COMMUNITY-BASED
PARTICIPATORY
RESEARCH

This book is dedicated to my husband Eric Menninger,
and my sons Elias and Nate

COMMUNITY-BASED
PARTICIPATORY
RESEARCH

KAREN HACKER

Institute for Community Health,
Cambridge Health Alliance, Harvard Medical School

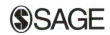

Los Angeles | London | New Delhi
Singapore | Washington DC

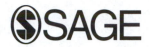

Los Angeles | London | New Delhi
Singapore | Washington DC

FOR INFORMATION:

SAGE Publications, Inc.
2455 Teller Road
Thousand Oaks, California 91320
E-mail: order@sagepub.com

SAGE Publications Ltd.
1 Oliver's Yard
55 City Road
London, EC1Y 1SP
United Kingdom

SAGE Publications India Pvt. Ltd.
B 1/I 1 Mohan Cooperative Industrial Area
Mathura Road, New Delhi 110 044
India

SAGE Publications Asia-Pacific Pte. Ltd.
3 Church Street
#10-04 Samsung Hub
Singapore 049483

Printed in the United States of America

Library of Congress Cataloging-in-Publication Data

A catalog record of this book is available from the Library of Congress.

9781452205816

This book is printed on acid-free paper.

Acquisitions Editor: Jerry Westby
Associate Editor: MaryAnn Vail
Production Editor: Brittany Bauhaus
Copy Editor: Kim Husband
Typesetter: Hurix Systems Pvt Ltd
Proofreader: Pam Suwinsky
Cover Designer: Gail Buschman
Marketing Manager: Lisa Sheldon-Brown
Permissions Editor: Karen Ehrmann

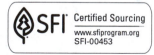

Certified Sourcing
www.sfiprogram.org
SFI-00453

14 15 16 10 9 8 7 6 5 4 3 2

Brief Contents

Detailed Contents

7. Conclusions

Prospectus

Community-Based Participatory Research

❖ MISSION OF THE TEXT

Research-based health care innovations make their way slowly, if at all, into community practice. It is the goal of community-based participatory research (CBPR) to create an effective translational process that will improve population health and increase connections with members of underserved communities.

Historically, research involving communities has not included community partners in a participatory manner. As a result, members of underserved communities often feel that research has been conducted upon them rather than with them. Rather than seeing potential community benefits from health care research in their communities, community members may feel exploited by researchers. The worst-case scenarios such as the Tuskegee experiment have left many communities, particularly those of color, feeling distrustful and reluctant to participate Consequently, research that has the potential to improve health may not result in action or sustainable change at the community level.

The CBPR approach seeks to improve the relevancy and acceptability of research and break down translational barriers. Members of underserved communities increasingly demand a new approach in which they are equal participants in the development and conduct of the research and in which the research has direct benefits for the people involved. CBPR aims to achieve these goals. In addition to health care, the CBPR approach is being used in education, psychology, and social work. In these various disciplines, community members are partnering with investigators who possess a variety of skills that will help improve the health and/or well-being of community members.

CBPR has been used successfully to help communities confront challenges ranging from youth suicide and violence to growing obesity trends.

This book was written to provide a succinct and easy-to-read practical guide to community-based participatory research. The book describes how an individual researcher might understand and then actually conduct CBPR research. It is thus a how-to book that uses case examples throughout. Both the benefits and challenges of the approach will be discussed, as well as the basic steps involved in CBPR projects. The book will also explore the unique ethical questions that arise in CBPR projects.

To date, comprehensive texts on CBPR are available but do not provide a practical guide to CBPR. Whereas other key texts cover the CBPR areas in depth, they do not offer a how-to approach to CBPR. With this book, students and teachers will have a short, easily accessible guide to CBPR that helps them as they consider and conduct CBPR in the field. It includes exercises at the end of each chapter with important take-home points. Additionally, this book will be available across a wide range of disciplines. The book will be seen primarily as a supplement for classes on research methods and substantive courses ranging from sociology to public health; it uses examples throughout emanating from the United States rather than Europe or Australia; it can be a valuable resource for both practitioners and community members.

❖ THE MARKET/COURSES FOR THE BOOK

The market for this book is diverse and includes students studying research methods in both the social sciences and medicine. The book could be used at either the undergraduate or graduate level in social work, sociology, psychology, education, public health, or medicine.

It might be helpful in the following types of courses:

Action research
CBPR, participatory research
Research methods
Evaluation
Community organizing
Clinical translational science

Professional organizations and journals that might have interest: American Public Health Association, Society of General Internal

Medicine, The National Institutes of Health Clinical Translational Science Awards, *American Journal of Public Health, Journal of General Internal Medicine, Journal of Preventive Medicine, Progress in Community Health Partnerships: Research, Education and Action, Clinical and Translational Science*, Community Campus Partnerships for Health, and community groups and organizations.

❖ THE MAJOR FEATURES OF THE BOOK AND
    BENEFITS OF THESE FEATURES

This book features short chapters that are clearly written in a "friendly," accessible manner that will appeal to beginners as well as community members while remaining sophisticated enough for researchers already involved in CBPR. Cases are interwoven throughout the chapters that help the reader apply the concepts that are outlined. In addition, basic tables are available to help visual learners and to summarize major concepts. Each chapter concludes with a set of activities for the classroom and, in some cases, questions for discussion. The chapter on the community perspective offers a perspective and practical concepts often overlooked in texts on the subject. The chapter on the steps in CBPR allows readers to get an understanding of steps in CBPR that can be practically applied in their own work. The book is also short enough to be seen as a supplement to other methods textbooks.

❖ THE SPECIAL PEDAGOGICAL AIDS AND
    HIGH-INTEREST FEATURES

Each chapter concludes with a set of questions and/or activities that are available for implementation in the classroom. CBPR is a participatory approach, and students need to experience and practice elements of the approach. When possible, it is advisable to attach field work to a CBPR course. Should this not be practical, exercises and activities that allow students to apply their knowledge in the classroom will be helpful.

❖ ACKNOWLEDGMENTS

I would like to acknowledge all the community partners that I have worked with throughout the years, in particular those that I have worked with in Somerville, Everett, and Cambridge who allowed their stories to be told in the book. Their commitment, advice, and perspectives have not only shaped the projects but also led to action-oriented outcomes. In addition, they have taught me enormous amounts about cultural humility, trust, and partnership. Their generosity of spirit and welcoming attitudes have been pivotal in my own development as a CBPR researcher. A number of specific individuals deserve mention, as they have greatly influenced the way that I think about CBPR. These include Alex Pirie and Milagro Grullon, who both provided quotes for the book. In addition, Milagro generously provided her insight to the community chapter. I would also like to thank the community members who participated in the 2010 conference titled Taking It to the Curbside: Engaging Communities to Create Sustainable Change for Health. Many of the quotes used in the book were from this conference.

I want to especially thank my colleagues at the Institute for Community Health: Dr. Justeen Hyde, Dr. Virginia Chomitz, Dr. Lise Fried, and Elisa Friedman. They have all been instrumental in shaping my understanding of CBPR and in refining our concepts. They have been my colleagues and friends in this pursuit and demonstrate their commitment and support to the communities we serve on a daily basis.

The Community Engaged Research subcommittee of the Harvard Catalyst Regulatory Core was helpful in defining the questions that were included in Chapter 6 on ethical considerations, as was Mr. Glover Taylor's assessment of the application of the Belmont principles to CBPR. I want to acknowledge the support of Dr. Russell Schutt, without whom I would not have been involved in developing this project.

I would also like to thank my editorial team at SAGE, Jerry Westby, publisher, and MaryAnn Vail, publishing associate, for all their hard work.

Most importantly, I want to thank my husband, Eric Menninger, and my two sons, Elias and Nate, who have been my support and strength throughout my career and the writing of this book. They have tolerated the many late-night community meetings and writing sessions, attended numerous community events, and provided my stability and inspiration.

1

Principles of Community-Based Participatory Research

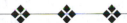

"Community-based participatory research is a collaborative research approach that is designed to ensure and establish structures for participation by communities affected by the issue being studied, representatives of organizations, and researchers in all aspects of the research process to improve health and well-being through taking action, including social change."[1]

In this chapter, I will provide an overview of community-based participatory research (CBPR) and accomplish the following objectives:

- Review the principles and foundations of CBPR
- Discuss the rationale for involvement in CBPR and when to use it (why bother?)

- Introduce cases in which CBPR was used to investigate
  - Policy issues
  - Urgent health crises
  - Health disparities
- Compare CBPR with traditional research
- Describe the strengths and weaknesses of a CBPR approach

❖ OVERVIEW OF COMMUNITY-BASED PARTICIPATORY RESEARCH

As is so often the case in community health practice, a problem is met head on with a solution. Unfortunately, while the solution represents a response to an urgent identified need, it often lacks an evidence base. We recognize that research-based innovations make their way slowly, if at all, into community practice.[2, 3] This has been documented extensively in the literature with regard to health in particular and speaks to the breakdown between academic and community-based practitioners. How can we speed the uptake of evidence into community practice? How can we identify the appropriate community-relevant research questions? How can we break down the barriers between researchers and community partners? How can communities translate their own practice-based evidence for consumption by the research community? There is a great deal of current interest in strategies to improve the rapidity of the translational research process.[4] Engaging the community may be one way to bridge the gap between science and practice.

Community-engaged research (CeNR) exists on a continuum ranging from research in the community setting to research that fully engages community partners. CBPR represents one end of this CeNR spectrum (Figure 1.1). The CBPR approach encourages engagement and full participation of community partners in every aspect of the research process from question identification to analysis and dissemination.

The goal of CBPR is to create an effective translational process that will increase bidirectional connections between academics and the communities that they study. This approach is not limited to specific disciplines but can be utilized whenever conducting community research. CBPR hinges on the relationship between the researcher and the community under study. The equitable aspects of the partnership and the participatory nature of the work differentiates CBPR from other traditional research approaches. In addition, in CBPR, there is a close linkage between the academic pursuit of generalizable knowledge and the use of that knowledge for action at the local level. Thus the practice of

Figure 1.1   Community-Engaged Research Continuum

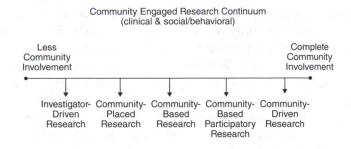

Source: Virginia Commonwealth University Center for Clinical and Translational Research 2008 (Looking at CBPR Through the Lens of the IRB. Cornelia Ramsey, PhD, MSPH Community Research Liaison, Center for Clinical and Translational Research, Division of Community Engagement, Department of Epidemiology & Community Health) http://www.research .vcu.edu/irb/Looking-at-CBPR-Through-the-Lens-of-the-IRB.ppt

CBPR takes a somewhat different track than that of traditional research. Throughout this chapter, I will focus on the rationale for CBPR, the principles, and the strengths and weaknesses of the approach in order to prepare the investigator to engage in CBPR projects.

Historically, research involving communities has not always included community partners in a participatory manner. Rather, research may be done in communities or on community residents, using the community as a laboratory. As a result, members of underserved communities often have negative perceptions of research and may feel exploited by investigators who conduct research, depart, and leave nothing behind. The worst-case scenarios such as the Tuskegee experiment have left many community members, particularly those of color, feeling distrustful and reluctant to participate in research.[5] Thus, research that may improve health and other outcomes may not include populations at highest risk or result in action or sustainable change at the community level.

In order to improve the relevancy and acceptability of research to communities and break down translational barriers, community members are increasingly demanding equality in the development and conduct of research. In addition, they are interested in shared ownership of the resulting data and in the application of results to action in practice or policy. In short, they want to have their voices heard and to participate in shaping the topics for study, identifying the emergent questions, and conducting investigations into the issues that are meaningful to their communities. They want to be part of the research team and see that the results are utilized to remedy problems at the community level.

Changing the research paradigm to include community members in a participatory manner requires a new approach that includes the formation of equitable partnerships between academia and community members in which there is mutual respect and both parties contribute and benefit. Thus, the goal of the CBPR approach is to produce research that is relevant to the life circumstances of communities and the people who reside within them.[6] When embraced by community partners as a shared endeavor, CBPR has the potential to catalyze actionable health improvement in real time.

❖ THE FOUNDATIONS OF CBPR

CBPR is only recently finding its way into the biomedical literature. However, it has been previously used in a variety of disciplines ranging from anthropology to education and psychology. Sometimes called "action research," "participatory research," "participatory action research,"[7] or even "street science,"[8] it has been used to examine environmental health issues, educational strategies, and international health issues.[9] These "participatory research" approaches share a core philosophy of inclusivity and of engaging the beneficiaries of research in the research process itself.[10] Similarly, CBPR is built on a foundation of social justice and empowerment, with its roots in feminist theory and community organizing. Feminist theory focuses on the historical and cultural oppression of women and drives toward gender equality and empowerment.[11] Community organizing purports that individuals together can make a difference in their own communities through group action.[12, 13] Both of these theories recognize that empowerment of the oppressed can result in community action for social change.

Two distinct traditions—that of Kurt Lewin, who coined the term *action research*, and that of Paulo Freire, who developed "emancipator research"—stand out as having influenced CBPR. Kurt Lewin in the 1940s was one of the first to use the term *action research*. Lewin sought to solve practical problems using a research cycle that involved planning, action, and investigation of the results of action.[7, 14] This iterative process paired the researcher with community members as partners in the investigative process. In 1970, Paulo Freire, the Brazilian educator, changed the power dynamics in research by depicting the researcher as facilitator and catalyst rather than director in his book, *Pedagogy of the Oppressed*.[15] As Freire noted, knowledge is connected to power—but whose power?

Knowledge does not only emanate from academia; rather, "people" also create and possess knowledge. This perspective shifts the concept of research from one in which the community is a laboratory for investigation to one in which community members not only participle in the inquiry process but also contribute their own knowledge. Freire framed the concept of "popular education" and argued that the teacher must be open to learning from the student. This colearning process based on emancipator conceptions has greatly influenced the use of CBPR approaches.[7]

In CBPR, the basic tenets of this participatory approach assume that there is knowledge and benefit in the shared partnership between academia and community. In *Street Science*, Corburn delineates where the power lies in the production of knowledge and highlights the value of local knowledge as an important component of the research process. In his examples, community members are the first to identify the question for study, and researchers are called to assist in solving real-world, practical problems[8] (Table 1.1).

Today, many view the CBPR process as iterative, similar to that described by Lewin. This allows the academic/community partnership to utilize data, refine programs, and ask additional questions. This is not unlike the Plan Do Study Act Cycle (PDSA) used in quality

Table 1.1   "Street Science": Where Is the Power in Knowledge Production?

Knowledge Production	Local Knowledge	Professional Knowledge
Who holds it?	Members of community—often identity group/place specific	Members of a profession, university, industry, government agency
How is it acquired?	Experience; interpersonal communication; cultural tradition	Experimental; epidemiologic; systematic data collection
What makes evidence credible?	Evidence of one's eyes, experience; personal communications	Often instrumentally mediated; statistical significance; legal standard
Forums where it is tested?	Public narratives; community stories, media	Peer review; courts; media

Source: Corburn, Jason., *Street Science: Community Knowledge and Environmental Health Justice*, Table 2.1, page 52, © 2005 Massachusetts Institute of Technology, by permission of The MIT Press.

Figure 1.2   Research for Process Improvement

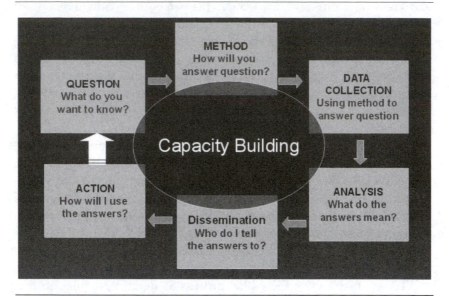

Source: Reproduced by permission from the Institute for Community Health, Cambridge, MA; 2011.

improvement (Figure 1.2). The systematic collection of data provides the community with opportunities for reflection, adjustment, and improvement in real time. CBPR offers access to data and skill sets that support this process. For example, in the following Everett example, community members observed an issue in their community that they wanted to address. Their question—Was the presence of Immigration and Customs Enforcement (ICE) impacting the health of the immigrant community?—required additional data. While they lacked the skills to conduct the investigation, they possessed an extensive knowledge of the community context, and they were invested in participating in the data collection, interpretation, and its ultimate use to shape local policy.

Example 1: Immigration: CBPR and Local Policy

In the last 20 years, Everett, Massachusetts, has seen an influx of immigrants coming from countries such as Brazil, Haiti, Guatemala, and Morocco. Everett is a small city of about 37,000 people with affordable rents and proximity to Boston. While there have been tensions in the community about issues related to immigration, such as housing and parking, it is only recently that the increased activity of Immigration and Customs Enforcement (ICE) has created challenges for the immigrant community. In particular, with increases in deportation and detention, immigrants fear that they will be picked up by authorities and deported. Stories of immigrants missing health appointments because ICE was in the vicinity or having stress-related conditions such as sleeplessness, headaches, and weight loss are common. These concerns were raised by various immigrant advocacy groups and Everett community leaders to institutional leaders. To facilitate changes in local policy, evidence was needed to support advocacy efforts and bring attention to the issue. So they approached a familiar academic partner to join them in an investigation of the problem, "the impact of ICE activity on immigrant health." Their goal was to learn more about the issue and solve the problem by developing a policy or programmatic intervention that would alleviate some of the stress that immigrants were experiencing.[16]

In the Everett CBPR project, the process started with a question that came from prior experience and community discourse. Community members wanted to validate their suspicions through rigorous methodology. Members approached a local researcher to assist them in their investigation, thus expanding their own skill sets. They were engaged in every step of the research process, including data collection. They ultimately took the results to action. Today, they are using the research for process-improvement cycles, asking additional questions, and sorting through methods with their academic partners to pursue new research projects.

❖ WHY BOTHER USING CBPR?

What are the forces driving us toward a CBPR approach? Today, as noted, there is an emerging realization that we must improve clinical translational research in order to improve human health.[17] CBPR holds promise as a strategy that would help to improve this process. Second, in the United States and abroad, we continue to have gross disparities in health outcomes. Minority racial/ethnic populations suffer disproportionately from many chronic disease conditions, and social determinants of health are heavily contributing to these disparities. Strategies for addressing these disparities require approaches that engage those most impacted in design and implementation. CBPR represents a promising approach to address these issues, as it relies on the community's self-determination of the research agenda and redistributes institutional resources into marginalized communities toward community benefit.[18]

There is also pressure from community partners who want to participate actively in research that involves them. They no longer want to be "laboratories" for research but, rather, they want to have access to data, solve their own local health and social issues, and drive policy. Community members want to conduct and participate in their own research endeavors. A CBPR approach validates this desire by not only including community members in all aspects of the research but also by building their capacity to lead and contribute to research projects. Simultaneously, it helps to build the capacity of academics to understand community context and improve the relevancy of their research. This colearning process is an important outcome of the CBPR approach.

❖ WHEN TO USE CBPR

A CBPR approach may be particularly useful for emergent problems for which community partners are in search of solutions but evidence is lacking. CBPR can be helpful in completing rapid assessments and as a strategy to engage hard-to-reach populations who may be less inclined to participate in research. And CBPR is exceptionally helpful in the formative phases of research when little is known about a topic area. CBPR helps academics understand the community perspective as they develop research questions and hypotheses together. Community partners can deepen the interpretation process once results are available, as they are intimately familiar with the context and meaning. Alternatively, CBPR is less likely to be helpful for study designs that require highly controlled methodology, as the participatory nature of the work tends to require flexibility and adaptation as part of the research process.

CBPR can be used when a specific issue emerges from the community and research partners are needed to rigorously assess the evidence and provide data. For example, CBPR has been used effectively for the study of environmental health issues. In some cases, CBPR is part of a real-time situation that demands answers and action. In others, it provides an important approach for understanding issues of vulnerable populations.

Example 2: Somerville: CBPR and Youth Suicide: Real-Time Health Crisis

Somerville, Massachusetts, is an urban city of 70,000 people that borders Cambridge. Historically, Somerville has been home to working-class populations, and in recent years, between gentrification and new immigration, the city demography has changed substantially. Somerville has also been affected by long-term substance abuse problems, especially heroin and alcohol. In 2001, a young person took his own life, and this was followed soon after by oxycodone overdoses of two high school students. A local researcher with an interest and experience in adolescent suicide was concerned that this might represent the beginning of a suicide cluster. She had prior relationships with community partners and so approached the Health Department director and mayor to discuss her concerns and interest.

Loss of youth life to suicide and overdose sends enormous ripples of concern through any community, and in Somerville, the Health and School Departments examined data from their biannual teen health survey to determine if suicidal behaviors had changed. The teen survey noted that 21% of the students had seriously considered suicide, and 14% had attempted suicide during the last 12 months. This was substantially elevated over previous years and higher than the state average overall.

In order to respond to the situation and investigate further, the mayor convened several task forces and asked the researcher to join with community members and colead one of the task forces along with the Health Department director. Other members included representation from the schools, the police, and community members as well as additional experts in suicide clusters. The questions posed by the community to the researcher were these:

- Was this suicide and overdose activity significantly elevated from baseline?
- Were there common links between victims and was this a contagion/cluster?

The overall aim of the partnership was to identify potential causes and strategies for action. In addition, the group wanted to establish a sustainable system that would effectively address the problem of suicide or additional crises in the long term.[19]

CBPR has also been used extensively to understand and explore health care disparities.[20] As per Dr. Wallerstein, CBPR has enhanced the effectiveness of interventions by integrating culturally based evidence and internal validity. In the following example, while the research question focused on disparities did not specifically come from the community, its application and acceptance were clearly driven by the perspectives of the community partners. And the ability to negotiate the investigation was grounded in a long-term academic/community partnership.

Example 3: BMI Disparities in Cambridge, Massachusetts

In Cambridge, Massachusetts, over a 10-year period, a coalition of school staff, public health personnel, and local researchers had been tracking childhood indicators of obesity. Using annual height and weight measurements of children that had been reported for many years, one researcher noted that there were glaring disparities in childhood obesity among racial/ethnic groups.[2] Blacks and Hispanics were carrying an undue burden of obesity. The researcher approached a long-time community colleague, and together they began to discuss the issue with other community members. The community colleague provided entrée to a social network of African American leaders and community members and helped engage them in conversation and the research process. Thus, the CBPR partnership expanded to include other members of the community, particularly the minority community, who came together to examine why disparities in obesity rates persisted even when general trends were declining (*Source:* Virginia R. Chomitz, Ph.D.,Tufts Medical School).

In this example, a CBPR approach provided inroads into important community voices that could lend meaning to the disparities identified. Without their understanding of the issue and participation in the research process, it would be unlikely that findings would be either relevant or valid for the population of concern.

❖   PRINCIPLES OF CBPR

The three examples described thus far illustrate many of the important principles of CBPR put forth by Dr. Barbara Israel and colleagues at the University of Michigan.[21] They are discussed below and described in greater detail elsewhere.[21, 22]

CBPR Acknowledges Community as a Unit of Identity

Understanding and identifying "the community" for the purposes of CBPR projects is an important first step in the CBPR process. Communities are made up of people linked by social ties who share common perspectives or interests and may also share a geographic location.[23] In our Everett example, the community was identified as "immigrants—documented and un-documented—living in Everett" and included the various community agencies (churches, immigrant advocacy groups, health and school departments, community organizations) that supported them. In our Somerville example, the community was identified as youth and youth-serving agencies throughout the city of Somerville. In our Cambridge example, the African American community was the focus.

CBPR Builds on Strengths and Resources Within the Community

In CBPR, the community as represented by its members, is a participant in the process and brings a variety of skill sets that are different than but equally as valuable as academic skills. Corburn refers to this knowledge as "street knowledge."[8] A community store owner, a pastor, a schoolteacher, a community member living in low-income housing understands community needs and the realities of daily life far better than a researcher does. In addition, the strengths of a given community can be brought to bear to implement solutions once identified. This offers the potential for sustainable change. As the action arm of CBPR, the community and its strengths play a particularly important role in carrying forward lessons learned. In all three of our examples, the community partners had a multiplicity of skill sets and "street knowledge" that was critical to the CBPR process. In Everett, community partners brought their extensive knowledge of the immigrant groups, including language skills and cultural experience. In Somerville, partners knew the history of the community and had intimate knowledge of the families who lost their children to substance abuse and suicide. In Cambridge, community partners provided access to diverse community members and leaders. In all three communities, the connections and social networks that community partners provided were the only avenues for academics to gain access to the population at risk and to understand the aftermath of losses. In addition, in all cases, community partners had the political and resource access necessary to ultimately translate findings into action.

CBPR Facilitates a Collaborative, Equitable Partnership in All Phases of Research, Involving an Empowering and Power-Sharing Process That Attends to Social Inequalities

CBPR hinges on the academic/community partnerships that are formed.[24] These partnerships are built on mutual respect and trust. Academics should recognize the inherent inequities that exist between community members and academics and try to address them via transparency, communication, shared decision making, and appropriate allocation of resources. In our examples, new partnerships were built on existing partnerships with a known researcher. The trust had, to some extent, already been built, thus opening the door for future projects. When the need arose, community partners were able to activate the partnership and participate from the beginning in all phases of the research, from identification of the problem to decisions about the methods and data collection.

CBPR Fosters Colearning and Capacity Building Among All Partners

One of the outcomes of a CBPR approach is the colearning that takes place by both community members and academics. As the academic learns of the community realities and the meaning of interactions from community members, so too the community members gain competencies in data use, critical thinking, and evaluation. All of this builds mutual capacity that will translate to other projects and enrich an understanding of community issues. As an example, in Everett, community partners identified the lack of driver's licenses as a major intervening factor in the relationship between ICE and immigrant health. That is, when an immigrant was stopped by police, the lack of a license led to arrest, and regardless of realities, immigrants believed that arrest by local police could lead to deportation. This was not something that the researchers were aware of. Similarly, the researchers actively educated the community partners on subjects ranging from how to develop a hypothesis to how to conduct focus groups.

CBPR Integrates and Achieves a Balance Between Knowledge Generation and Intervention for the Mutual Benefit of All Partners

CBPR is nested in real-world issues, and the relevant problems of interest demand action. Balancing the demands of community action with the needs of research can be challenging. Pacing may differ, analytic methods may clash, and dissemination efforts may conflict. When the CBPR process works best, it can satisfy both needs. These issues should be discussed up front and frequently throughout the process so that difficult issues can be effectively navigated. In our Somerville example, in the midst of a crisis, community members wanted and demanded action. Researchers provided information on existing evidence-based practices for their adoption, including the Centers for Disease Control and Prevention (CDC) recommendations. They also were instrumental in collecting and mapping data in an ongoing manner. In this case, knowledge generation and interventions were happening simultaneously, and while the balance was achieved to some extent, it was necessary to prioritize action given the urgency of the situation.

CBPR Focuses on the Local Relevance of Public Health Problems and on Ecological Perspectives That Attend to the Multiple Determinants of Health

The problems explored in CBPR studies are generally of great relevance to the communities involved. As such, CBPR necessarily will involve the "social determinants" as important factors to be considered and explored.

The examples offered were not only relevant to community public health problems but also took a larger perspective, recognizing that the external conditions had much to do with the issues under study. These types of projects demand multidisciplinary teams of community members and scientists. In Everett, we worked with lawyers, demographers, and physicians as well as immigrant leaders, clergy, and local government officials, all of whom contributed their knowledge to the process.

CBPR Involves Systems Development Using a Cyclical and Iterative Process

CBPR is often perceived as a cyclical process involving numerous phases from question development to data collection and analysis. As with the quality-improvement cycles used in health care improvement and business (Plan Do Study Act), the process often opens the door to new and emerging questions, which in turn requires an investigative process.

In all of our examples, initial data collection and analysis sparked new lines of inquiry. As data became available during the suicide crisis, community members sought to explore and answer these new questions: that is, were these suicides related to drug use? In addition, they used the data to refine their interventions, including educational efforts and outreach to subpopulations within the community. In the Cambridge example, data that had been collected over time (BMI data) focused on the entire school-aged population, but further examination of this data sparked a whole new line of inquiry: that of disparities in obesity rates.

CBPR Disseminates Results to All Partners and Involves Them in the Wider Dissemination of Results

The dissemination process in CBPR is somewhat different than that typically used in traditional research endeavors. Dissemination needs to benefit all parties and means different things to academics than it does to community partners. For example, dissemination from a community perspective may require different formats and venues than the peer-reviewed journal. In addition, the time sequencing may be different, as there is often a more rapid demand for results at the community level than in academic realms. Thus, negotiating types of dissemination and what can be disseminated when, is an important element in CBPR work. In Everett, dissemination took the form of a community forum that presented the data back to members of the affected community for their consideration. In Somerville, dissemination was happening in an ongoing manner throughout the project. However, ultimately, all the partners were involved in developing a final synopsis of the work. This ended up as a peer-reviewed paper aimed at providing information for other communities that might encounter similar events.[19] Similarly, in Cambridge, the data were used both for a report to the community and the advisory group and for a peer-reviewed paper.

CBPR Involves a Long-Term Process and Commitment to Sustainability

To fully engage in CBPR, the researcher needs to consider the time involved for specific projects but also to nurture relationships outside of projects. How do researchers get to know their partners? How much time is spent in the community at nonwork events? Do they make the long-term commitment to improving the community situation, or is this a "one-shot" research project? In order to establish the trust needed to fully engage in CBPR, a long-term commitment will likely extend beyond the specific project to other worthy projects that partners feel are appropriate.

❖ CBPR VS. TRADITIONAL RESEARCH

CBPR changes the power dynamics inherent in traditional research. Researchers are typically seen as the experts and in possession of knowledge. In CBPR, the community members possess knowledge and are experts in community context, norms, and issues. CBPR attempts to establish equitable partnerships with mutual responsibility. This is in direct contrast to more traditional forms of research (Table 1.2) in which the investigator leads and is responsible for both the conduct and outcomes of the process. For example, where traditional research identifies the question of interest, in CBPR, community partners are the initiators of the research question.

Table 1.2   Differences Between Traditional Research and Community-Engaged Research

	Community-Engaged Research	
Traditional research approach	*Research with the community*	*Community-based participatory research approach*
Researcher defines problem	Research IN the community or WITH the community	Community identifies problem or works with researcher to identify the problem
Research IN or ON the community	Research WITH community as partner	Research WITH community as full partner
People as subjects	People as participants	People as participants and collaborators
Community organizations may assist	Community organizations may help recruit participants and serve on advisory board	Community organizations are partners with researchers
Researchers gain skills and knowledge	Researchers gain skills and knowledge, some awareness of helping community develop skills	Researcher and community work together to help build community capacity
Researchers control process, resources, and data interpretation	Researchers control research; community representatives may help make minor decisions	Researcher and community share control equally
Researchers own data and control use and dissemination	Researchers own the data and decide how they will be used and disseminated	Data are shared, researchers and community decide how they will be used and disseminated

Source: From "Practicing Community Engaged Research," © 2007 by Mary Anne McDonald, MA, DrPH. Duke Center for Community Research, Dept of Community and Family Medicine, Duke University Medical Center, Durham, NC 27710. Adapted from Community Campus Partnerships for Health on-line curriculum: Developing and Sustaining Community-Based Participatory Research Partnerships: A Skill Building Curriculum (http://www.ccph.info/)

Whether initiators or collaborators, the study question will need to be of interest to both the researcher and the community partners. Concepts of collaboration, equity, power sharing, and consensus are all elemental to CBPR. Research with rather than on the community is the focus, and the participatory nature of the process requires investigators to be attuned to the perspectives of community partners. These differences in approach are well illustrated in our examples, where community partners and researchers were engaged in a partnership to address the research questions.

❖ STRENGTHS AND WEAKNESSES OF CBPR

Now that you are familiar with the "what" and "why" of CBPR, it is important to also understand the strengths and limitations of this approach (Table 1.3). CBPR is likely to facilitate more relevant research given its community-embedded nature. Community input may reveal information that would have been otherwise undiscovered and that potentially greatly enhances the research process and the results. This additional value encourages community ownership and may support sustainability. CBPR also helps build community and researcher capacity to understand and utilize data and to think critically about impact and outcomes. For example, in Everett, the findings from the immigrant study were used to establish police/immigrant dialogue and change local policy related to traffic stops. Local police no longer arrested people for lacking driver's licenses but, rather, issued citations instead, which substantially decreased fear in the immigrant community. The acquisition of new skills and access to resources for community partners are also benefits of the CBPR process. In Somerville, community members learned mapping techniques and continued to monitor 911 data on overdoses and suicide as part of health department responsibilities. CBPR is also likely to improve participation and retention in studies, particularly for populations that are unlikely to be involved in research. This was certainly true in the Everett study, in which more than half the participants in the study were undocumented immigrants. Other studies have identified recruitment and retention as major benefits of CBPR, particularly important for research on disparities.[1]

As partnerships deepen, CBPR may effectively blur the separation between academic researchers and community partners. Members of marginalized communities embark on an investigative process to

Table 1.3   Strengths and Weaknesses of a CBPR Approach

Strengths	Weaknesses
Relevancy to local community (authenticity)	Time needed to form partnerships
Community ownership	Potential loss of control
Builds local capacity and community skills	May not be generalizable (external validity)
Builds researcher skills	Requires flexibility given changes in contextual factors
Builds trust and bridges community academic barriers	Time frames for reporting results may differ
Supports social action	Conflict between partners on dissemination, strategies, decisions
Imparts in-depth knowledge of community context, needs, and assets	May impact method choice
Deepens interpretation of results	May not be valued in academic environment
Results directly used for sustainable changes	

understand their own circumstances through the systematic collection of data. They become researchers themselves. So, too, as the researchers engage in CBPR, they will gain a whole new set of skills that stems from their understanding of appropriate language, methods, meaning, and context. These skills and enhanced knowledge of community needs and assets will lead to improved validity and value of their projects. It is this transformative process that builds colearning and mutual respect within the partnership.

However, CBPR also has it challenges. A major weakness from a researcher perspective is that CBPR takes time: time to build relationships with partners, time to manage a participatory group, and time beyond specific projects to maintain partnerships.[25] This is unlikely to be compensated by academic institutions. In addition, given that the contextual environment is constantly changing, there may be difficulties maintaining partnerships as priorities shift and personnel change within the community. For example, if you are working with a mayor and local leadership and the mayor loses an election, you may be faced with developing new partnerships with different leaders to continue the work.

A participatory approach also requires an academic partner to be flexible, creative, and able to facilitate group processes. Given that decision making is shared and plans may change, these attributes are important in the conduct of CBPR. For example, should a new issue emerge in the community under study, it may be hard to maintain focus on the research initiative, as partners may divert their attention elsewhere. You may be working on asthma-related environmental issues when a local leader becomes a victim of violence. In response, the community members turn their attention toward the new, pressing issue, which takes precedent. This forces an unexpected slowdown in the project.

The participatory process also forces potential compromises in research design. For example, the researcher may want the strongest design, such as randomization of participants to test an educational intervention, but community partners feel that they do not want to limit access to any new educational resource regardless of whether it is proven effective. Randomization may therefore be considered unethical in a school environment. In another situation, community partners may be concerned that implementing a research protocol in a busy youth program does not work well with the delivery of service. They may restrict access to clients or limit the amount of information that can be obtained. Overall, given that decision making is shared, research design must be negotiated and determined feasible by the community under investigation.

One of the major issues raised regarding CBPR is that given its local focus, can it be generalizable to other environments? That is, do CBPR studies have sufficient external validity?[20] While CBPR tends to be used at the local level, generalizable validity (external validity) is dependent on how conclusions drawn from one community can be translated to other communities. Much of this question is dependent on how well the investigators were able to limit bias, on how "comparable" other communities might actually be, and most importantly, on how well community partners are able to adapt the research to meet their needs and unique assets. Each community exists in a frame of contextual variables that can range from population demographics to a host of contextual factors, including local politics, regulations, physical environment, and so on. These make it difficult to strictly transfer the knowledge learned in one community to others. While achieving external validity is challenging in CBPR, it can be done, and I will address methods in a later chapter.

The CBPR process also requires negotiation and compromise. Researchers must develop listening skills. Data and results are products of a shared enterprise, which requires an agreed upon set of rules. I will discuss partnership building and management in a later chapter.

While there are numerous challenges inherent in CBPR partnerships, it is the very process of working through these challenges that makes the projects and partnerships stronger, builds community capacity, enhances investigator skills, and empowers community partners. The process of colearning benefits all involved and yields important findings for direct application to real-life situations.

❖ CONCLUSION

CBPR is an approach that engages the community under study in every aspect of the research process. In so doing, it improves the relevancy and appropriateness of research. It encourages a team approach to some of the world's most immutable problems and helps to translate research into practical, real-world interventions. The foundational underpinnings of the approach from Lewin to Freire discuss the need to develop equitable meaningful partnerships to meet these goals. There are challenges to doing CBPR, but there are many benefits. Over the course of this book, we will help the reader understand the major steps in doing CBPR. We hope the reader will consider when and how to use CBPR and that this approach will be benefit communities nationwide.

❖ QUESTIONS AND ACTIVITIES

Activities

Invite a local community partner to join the class discussion and provide his or her perspective on research. Then have students break up into discussion groups to identify the challenges and benefits of a CBPR approach to research.

Have students read a CBPR study and provide a critique of the strengths and weaknesses of the approach for the problem under study.

Questions for Discussion

1. How does CBPR challenge and contribute to the fundamental constructs of research?

2. What is the benefit of identifying and using local knowledge?

3. What are the potentially conflicting agendas of communities and academics?

4. What are some of the challenges inherent in CBPR?

5. Discuss the threats to external validity when using a CBPR approach. Brainstorm strategies for improving external validity when working with community partners.

❖ NOTES

1.   Viswanathan M, Ammerman A, Eng E, Gartlehner G, Lohr KN, Griffith D, Rhodes S, Samuel-Hodge C, Maty S, Lux, L, Webb L, Sutton SF, Swinson T, Jackman A, Whitener L. *Community-Based Participatory Research: Assessing the Evidence.* Evidence Report/Technology Assessment No. 99 (Prepared by RTI–University of North Carolina Evidence-based Practice Center under Contract No. 290-02-0016). AHRQ Publication 04-E022-2. Rockville, MD: Agency for Healthcare Research and Quality; 2004:22.

2.   Szilagyi PG. Translational research and pediatrics. *Academic Pediatrics.* 2009 Mar-Apr;9(2):71–80.

3.   Heller C, de Melo-Martin I. Clinical and translational science awards: can they increase the efficiency and speed of clinical and translational research? *Academic Medicine.* 2009 Apr;84(4):424–32.

4.   Glasgow RE, Emmons KM. How can we increase translation of research into practice? Types of evidence needed. *Annual Review of Public Health.* 2007 Jan 1;28:413–33.

5.   Corbie-Smith G, Thomas SB, St George DM. Distrust, race, and research. *Archives of Internal Medicine.* 2002 Nov 25;162(21):2458–63.

6.   Horowitz CR, Robinson M, Seifer S. Community-based participatory research from the margin to the mainstream: are researchers prepared? *Circulation: Journal of the American Heart Association.* 2009;119:2633–42.

7.   Wallerstein N, Duran B. The theoretical, historical, and practice roots of CBPR. In: Minkler M, Wallerstein N, eds. *Community-Based Participatory Research for Health.* 2nd ed. San Francisco, CA: Jossey-Bass; 2008:26–46.

8.   Corburn J. *Street Science: Community Knowledge and Environmental Health Justice.* Cambridge, MA: MIT Press; 2005.

9. Minkler M, Wallerstein N., eds. *Community-Based Participatory Research for Health*. San Francisco: Jossey-Bass; 2003.

10. Cargo M, Mercer SL. The value and challenges of participatory research: strengthening its practice. *Annual Review of Public Health*. 2008 April;29:325–50.

11. Devault M, Ingraham C. Metaphors of silence and voice in feminist thought. In: Devault M, ed. *Liberating Method*. Philadelphia, PA: Temple University Press; 1999:175–86.

12. Bobo K, Kendall J, Max S. *Organizing for Social Change*. 3rd ed. Santa Ana, CA: Seven Locks Press; 2001.

13. Chambers E, Cowan MA. *Roots for Radicals: Organizing for Power, Action, and Justice*. New York: Continuum International Publishing Group; 2003.

14. Lewin K. *Resolving Social Conflicts and Field Theory in Social Science*. Washington, DC: American Psychological Association; 1997.

15. Freire P. *Pedagogy of the Oppressed*. New York, NY: Continuum International; 1970.

16. Hacker K, Chu J, Leung C, Marra R, Pirie A, Brahimi M, English M, Beckmann J, Acevedo-Garcia D, Marlin RP. The impact of Immigration and Customs Enforcement on immigrant health: perceptions of immigrants in Everett, Massachusetts, USA. *Social Science & Medicine*. 2011 Aug;73(4):586–94.

17. Heller C, de Melo-Martin I. Clinical and translational science awards: can they increase the efficiency and speed of clinical and translational research? *Academic Medicine*. 2009 Apr;84(4):424–32.

18. Minkler M. Linking science and policy through community-based participatory research to study and address health disparities. *American Journal of Public Health*. 2010 Apr 1;100 Suppl 1:S81–87.

19. Hacker K, Collins J, Gross-Young L, Almeida S, Burke N. Coping with youth suicide and overdose: one community's efforts to investigate, intervene, and prevent suicide contagion. *Crisis*. 2008;29(2):86–95.

20. Wallerstein N, Duran B. Community-based participatory research contributions to intervention research: the intersection of science and practice to improve health equity. *American Journal of Public Health*. 2010 Apr 1;100 Suppl 1:S40–46.

21. Israel BA, Eng E, Schulz AJ, Parker EA, eds. Introduction to methods in community-based participatory research for health. In Israel BA, Eng E, Schulz AJ, Parker EA, eds. *Methods in Community-Based Participatory Research for Health*. San Francisco, CA: Jossey-Bass; 2005:2–26

22. Wallerstein NB, Duran B. Using community-based participatory research to address health disparities. *Health Promotion Practice*. 2006 Jul;7(3):312–23.

23. MacQueen KM, McLellan E, Metzger DS, Kegeles S, Strauss RP, Scotti R, Blanchard L, Trotter RT. What is community? An evidence-based definition for participatory public health. *Ameican Journal of Public Health*. 2001 Dec;91(12):1929–38.

24. Christopher S, Watts V, McCormick AK, Young S. Building and maintaining trust in a community-based participatory research partnership. *American Journal of Public Health*. 2008 Aug;98(8):1398–406.

25. Norris K, Brusuelas R, Jones L, Miranda J, Duru O, Mangione C. Partnering with community-based organizations: an academic institution's evolving perspective. *Ethnicity & Disease*. 2007 Winter;17(1 Suppl 1):S27–32.

2

Defining the Community and Power Relationships

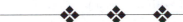

"Reviews of the effectiveness of collaborations for improving community health indicate that they can be effective but that there are many potential obstacles to realizing the benefits of a participatory approach in both public health research and programs. In particular, the lack of an accepted definition of community can result in different collaborators forming contradictory or incompatible assumptions about community and can undermine our ability to evaluate the contribution of community collaborations to achievement of public health objectives."[1]

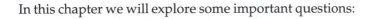

In this chapter we will explore some important questions:

- What is community?
- Who represents community?
- What is a community advisory board?
- Who are the right stakeholders?

- What are the existing power relationships between academics and community partners?
- What are the rules of CBPR partnerships?
- What are strategies for assessing community readiness for research?

❖ WHAT IS COMMUNITY?

When embarking on a CBPR project, one of the first challenges is to define the community of interest. Who is the population of interest? What are the boundaries of their "community"? Is this a community that is geographically bounded (city, neighborhood, county) or one that is nongeographically defined by a common culture (Latinos, African Americans) or condition (parents of children with special needs) or other shared concern? Are you planning to work with those directly impacted by the issue or with the organizations that represent or serve them? The CBPR approach is often used to examine issues for under-served populations, to give voice to their concerns and help identify their perspective on the problem. However one chooses to define "community," it remains the conceptual underpinning of CBPR, influencing who collaborates and participates, how sampling is conducted, where dissemination takes place, and, most importantly, how relevant the work is to the community of interest.

Example 1: Everett Immigrant Health

A community coalition in Everett was interested in engaging a researcher to learn more about the health implications of Immigration and Customs Enforcement (ICE) on immigrant health in their community. The coalition had a diverse membership, including agency directors, school administrators, several teachers, and representatives from several immigrant advocacy groups. Many were leaders in local Everett institutions (schools, community-based organizations). They had come together previously around a multiplicity of health and social service issues and together had successfully garnered resources for new programming. They shared common interests in wanting to make a difference in their city. While they generally defined their "community" as geographic—that is, those who worked and lived in Everett—they were particularly concerned with the most vulnerable populations (e.g., the poor, recent immigrants, and youth). Thus, for the CBPR project, they defined community as Everett, Massachusetts, but more specifically, as the underserved population of recent immigrants and, in particular, immigrants who were undocumented.

The term *community* has many meanings throughout the social sciences.[2] Hillery (1955) identified more than 90 different definitions of *community* in prior literature.[3] The majority of authors, however, consistently cite certain characteristics in their definitions, including social interaction, geographic area, and common ties.[1] Anthropology, sociology, public health, and psychology have all looked at communities slightly differently. Even within a discipline, there is no consistent agreement on the definition. Cultural anthropology tends to take an ethnographic perspective of community, examining the structure, norms, and social mores that bind individuals together.[4] Sociology builds upon the concept of social capital and the interconnectedness of community members.[5] Public health identifies the social and political responsibility of community and sees the community as a population. Psychology brings up the concepts of "a sense of community" and shared emotional connection.[9-11] All of these elements are part of our understanding of "community" (Table 2.1).

Table 2.1   Examples of Key Constructs in Defining "Community"

MacQueen[1]	Joint action	Locus	Sharing common interests and perspectives	Social ties	Diversity of communities within communities
Hillery[3]	Social integration	Geographic area		Common ties	
McKeown[4]	Shared action	Locality	Common institutions	Biological and social membership	Diverse characteristics of members
Chavis and Newbrough[6]	Influence	Fulfillment of need	Shared emotional connection	Membership	
Patrick and Wickizer[7]	Social interaction	Place	Social and political responsibility	Members who share concerns in communal groupings	Diverse communities that change over time
Wellman and Wortley[8]	Social support	Social support networks	Social interaction and support	Social support ties	Diverse types of support (kinship neighbors, friends, organizations)

Thus, as we think about community and working with communities, we may consider different ways of realizing the concept. For example, many define community by its geographic and political boundaries (city, county), while others may consider it any group of people that share a common set of characteristics (immigrants, women, parents). *Community* can also refer to a group of people bound together by shared condition or concern, such as a community of diabetics or a community of parents with children who have special needs. MacQueen and colleagues conducted a series of interviews to determine what community meant and identified a common definition that works well: *a group of people with diverse characteristics who are linked by social ties, share common perspectives, and engage in joint action in geographical locations or settings.*[1] However, more importantly, she found that different groups had slightly different definitions about how they saw their communities. Today, with the advent of the Internet and social networking, communities cross geographic boundaries as well as age, gender, and race/ethnicity. As these tools become more and more popular, we need to broaden our definitions of community beyond physical geography.[12] Wellman and Wortley have argued that community locus is less important and that "personal networks" are better used in defining community.[8] There may be multiple communities within communities, and individuals may be members of multiple communities.

When the term *community* is used, it often assumes homogeneity, singularity, cohesiveness, and consensus: what community X wants or what community Y believes. In fact, no community is homogeneous; there will always be a diversity of ideas, beliefs, and even communities within communities. In CBPR, it is important to recognize the diversity of community and learn from its members how it is defined and conceptualized. Recognizing how you are operationalizing your definition of "community" for the purposes of a CBPR project is the first step in your process. And your definition of community will also influence what the research project may or may not do or show for that community.

Once identified, the process of learning about a community is a pivotal task for the CBPR researcher. This takes time. It is an exploration that involves gathering existing and new data, meeting individuals and groups, building relationships, assessing strengths and weaknesses, and learning about the culture. To gain this knowledge, the researcher needs to spend time in the community learning about the existing social networks and the community institutions, organizations, and coalitions. The researcher needs to become familiar with the formal and informal leaders who can also provide insight into the political landscape and provide entrée into the community of interest. For those interested in pursuing CBPR, it is best to develop these relationships prior to launching a research project. Showing up at meaningful community events, having coffee with community members outside of work hours, or visiting organizations and sitting down with their directors are all ways of building relationships and demonstrating your commitment to the community that will be appreciated by your community partners. This process will help the researcher decide who to approach in the community engagement process and provides the foundation for the academic/community research partnership. In addition, through this "getting to know the community" process, the researcher should start to understand and map out the community strengths and assets.

❖ WHO REPRESENTS COMMUNITY?

In CBPR, there is tacit agreement that "community" should include those impacted by the research issue[13]—that is, those patients, community members, and residents who are impacted by the issue under study. However, it is challenging to think about engaging community members, one individual at a time. Unless you have extensive community organizing skills, this can be a difficult challenge. Rather, many who conduct CBPR will work with organizations that represent the community of interest or with communities that have some organizational structure (representative leadership). This might include community coalitions, community-based organizations, advocacy groups, or local institutions such as schools, mayors' offices, or health care providers. Both strategies can work well in CBPR; however, this author believes that while a participatory approach may be utilized with any group of interested community members, a CBPR project that does not elicit the experience of those impacted by the problem under study does not fully meet the goals of CBPR.

This brings us to the question of who represents community in a CBPR project. While working with institutions (government, community-based organizations, churches, and their leaders) provides the infrastructure necessary to forge CBPR relationships and conduct

Table 2.2   Questions to Consider in Community Group Engagement

Does this community group have representation of the population of interest?	*Is the membership stable? Is the leadership engaged?*
Does this group have long-standing ties to the community?	*How long has the group existed? What's their reputation? Can they get things done?*
Do they have the ability to outreach to the population of interest or the community at large?	*Have they done outreach before? Does their staff have experience and success with outreach?*
Do they have adequate infrastructure to participate in partnership?	*Can they enter into contracts? Are they incorporated? Have they done CBPR before? Can they manage grants?*

research, these organizations have differing abilities to represent the community voice. The experience will be quite different than working with a grassroots organization or a community coalition. A CBPR investigator needs to be aware of the strengths and limitations of working with different types of community groups and/or institutions. Important questions to ask of the group you choose to partner with are noted in Table 2.2.

The CBPR investigator also needs to understand the strengths and limitations of the representatives at the table. Israel and colleagues note that participatory approaches that rely on choosing representatives of community can be fraught with potential conflicts.[14] Often, community leaders are identified as the representatives of the community, and while they have an understanding from their vantage point about the community, they may or may not be viewed by the populace as appropriate representatives. It is impossible to achieve full community representation in CBPR, but learning about the community and identifying leaders is a process. Constructing a community advisory group to facilitate representation is one strategy used in many CBPR projects.

❖ THE COMMUNITY ADVISORY BOARD AND MEMBERSHIP

CBPR requires community participation. Participation requires a structured relationship with community partners so that members can engage throughout the project. Working with a "community advisory board" (CAB) is one way that an investigator can interface with community members and maintain an open dialogue.[15-18] The CAB can act in an advisory role for multiple projects,[15] or it can function as the community members of the research team for one project. It can be fluid or rigorously constructed with elected or appointed members, depending on partner preferences. How does this CAB get established? In some cases, such as in our Everett example, the advisory group was ready-made. There was an informal coalition of concerned leaders who approached the researcher. Their collaboration was based in previous activities including a Multicultural Affairs Commission. As their coalition evolved, they added leaders from different institutions (schools, after-school programs, churches) and additional members to fill in perceived gaps and expand the diversity of their membership. The following describes members of the Everett advisory group; these representatives joined the research team for the duration of the immigrant project.

"Six Everett community agencies, many members of the MAC, who had been actively involved in addressing immigrant issues in Everett, were involved in the research project: the Joint Committee for Children's Health Care in Everett (JCCHCE), the Everett Literacy Program, the Muslim American Civic and Cultural Association (MACCA), Immaculate Conception and St. Anthony's Catholic churches, La Comunidad, Inc., and the Everett police department. The JCCHCE focuses its efforts on improving access to health care and is actively involved in enrollment in both insurance and in the state Health Care Safety Net program.[19] The two Catholic churches' congregations include large numbers of Haitians and Brazilians. La Comunidad and MACCA are emerging immigrant service organizations focused on Latinos and the Arab and Muslim population respectively and both are led by immigrants. The Everett Literacy Program provides the majority of English Second Language courses in Everett. Representatives from these groups had extensive experience in coalition building, community organizing, and addressing immigrant concerns."[20]

Unfortunately, an existing activated coalition or the "right" coalition is not always available or interested in partnering. It is often incumbent on the investigator to make contacts, develop relationships, and assess potential partners toward convening their own CAB. As investigators get to know the community, they may find that there are smaller groups of community members who want to work on an issue. There may be community activists who have strong opinions and want action. In every community, there are the go-to individuals, who may be formal or informal leaders. Their ability to organize community members and facilitate CBPR is a critical asset; however, it is equally important to understand their role in the political matrix of the community. In short, it is important to know whether they have clout and whether they have access to the community of interest.

Example 2: Somerville Youth Suicides and Overdoses

In the midsized urban community of Somerville, Massachusetts, there was a suicide cluster that affected young people over the course of a 5-year period. During this crisis, the mayor brought together a task force—the Mayor's Suicide and Mental Health Task Force— that included many of his department heads (schools, police, health department), leaders of local youth-serving agencies, health organizations, mental health and substance abuse organizations, and a CBPR research organization. Many of these leaders did not live in Somerville or had short-term histories in the city, and they did not have direct connections to the population at highest risk. It was important to add representation from long-standing community members who knew the families and the children. Several community activists became involved in the task force, and they were able to reach out to those most at risk in a way that was impossible for many of the professionals involved. These informal leaders acted as connectors between the professionals and academics and the population at risk. Finding these individuals can be a challenge, but their contribution to CBPR efforts is invaluable.[21]

In establishing a CAB, both the investigator and the community partners need to ask whether the current representatives are the "right" representatives. Any community group wishing to engage in CBPR should do a self-assessment to determine if the right people are part of the process. The investigator may not have the in-depth knowledge of the community to make this determination. Here is where community insight provides guidance to identify the appropriate membership for a CAB. They know who the players are and understand how to avoid the political minefields. The strength of their relationships in the community will benefit the CBPR project, as they can utilize their own social networks to engage other community members. In our Everett example, we added several new members to the research team, including youth and immigrant leaders, to help us access the populations of interest. These individuals were invited by CAB members who were building on their existing relationships. In CBPR, existing social networks are a powerful tool for community engagement.[12]

❖ POWER DYNAMICS

"What is important and interesting for me is how you enter a partnership. The transparency principle is key but it's difficult because the community does not like the word research. But it's important to be open about this and say that I'm an academic. It's important [that] the agenda of the researchers are known" (Community partner-conference participant).[22]

"Trust is not something you hand to people. You have to earn it." (Community partner-conference participant)[22]

Elements of successful partnerships include power sharing, open communication, equitable division of labor and resources, and mutual recognition.[23] Partnerships are based on mutual respect and trust. Building partnerships is a challenging endeavor, especially since academics and community partners may differ dramatically in their professional experiences, their access to resources, their research literacy, and their comfort level in the community. The power and privilege connected with race, class, and educational attainments may be a wedge that separates the investigator from the community.[24] The researcher may be associated with unearned advantages just by being affiliated with an academic institution or by having letters after his or her name. This is particularly true for communities that have been historically marginalized with deeply rooted experiences of discrimination and disadvantage. Throughout history, there are examples of unethical research that has impacted disadvantaged and minority populations, leaving a legacy of mistrust and disappointment. In addition, communities have experienced years of "being studied" by universities who don't give back.

"Communities have no motivation because these research projects go on yet there is no investment in the community after...." (Community partner-conference participant)[22]

The academic/community conflicts of long standing are played out in town/gown politics and exemplified by ivory tower mentalities. Academic institutional resources, whether real or perceived, are generally unavailable to the community. Thus, while CBPR is rooted in social justice and requires "collaborative, equitable partnerships" that "promote co-learning and capacity building among partners,"[14] dealing with power and privilege can present critical challenges in the CBPR process.[24] Researchers must ask themselves about their own commitment and capabilities to engage in a CBPR project. Do they possess the skills and knowledge that will enable them to be effective partners?

How do we negotiate the inherent power dynamics of academic community partnerships? Respect and trust are not automatic. Investigators need to get to know the community. They need to spend time just "showing up" at events unrelated to the research. They need to be collaborative in their approach and humble in their demeanor. The term *cultural humility*, coined by Tervalon and Murray-Garcia (1998), refers to "a process that requires humility as individuals continually engage in self-reflection and self-critique as lifelong learners...."[25] While *cultural humility* was initially applied in the realm of clinical care, it can be applied to CBPR. Investigators involved in CBPR need to assess their own cultural beliefs and assumptions in order to address power imbalances and develop partnerships based in mutual trust.[24] They need to listen and demonstrate their commitment to the community long before and after the actual project begins. Then they need to negotiate the research agenda with their partners in an equitable manner that extends from decisions about design to those about budgetary concerns. Throughout the process, they need to be transparent. You may never be able to completely erase the historical experiences or the reality of resources, but through the practice of cultural humility and by explaining the situation to your partners from the beginning, you are more likely to build the trusting relationships that are needed for successful CBPR. Building partnerships is a long-term commitment that can take years.

"While this person is a community member that may not have a Ph.D., they have input that is just as equally important and applicable." (Community partner-conference participant)[22]

In Somerville, as a researcher, my most important mentor was a community activist who had grown up in Somerville and owned the local tattoo parlor. She knew the families and peers of the young people who had committed suicide. She warned me not to try to go directly to the young people to do the investigation of the suicides. She said I would be perceived as a privileged outsider who was going to tell them they had mental health problems. Instead, she urged me to work with her to create a conduit to these youth. This was very difficult, as I thought myself an expert in the field. But her advice proved critical as we addressed the problems in the community. She was a trusted insider who was able to act as a liaison between the affected community and the professionals.

As with any relationship, CBPR partnerships depend on mutual trust, credibility, and strong personal relationships. Practicing and demonstrating cultural humility, a willingness to share power, to engage in collaborative decision making, to show up, and to demonstrate your commitment to the community after the specific research project is over are all important lessons in CBPR.

❖ COMMUNITY READINESS FOR RESEARCH

As part of building a CBPR partnership, there are many considerations that both community partners and researchers should consider prior to and throughout the engagement process. A pre–CBPR assessment can help both parties avoid pitfalls during the study itself. Table 2.3 notes the list of questions that should be considered before engaging in CBPR. Answering these questions will help both parties understand the challenges and benefits of participation. In particular, as part of the development of a partnership pre–CBPR, community members should ask several specific questions to assess their own readiness for research. Do they have the time to participate without sacrificing their other responsibilities? Are they going to get appropriate financial resources to support their work from the researcher? Do they have

Table 2.3   Readiness for CBPR

Questions for community partners to ask researcher prior to engaging in CBPR

1. What kind of partnership does the researcher have in mind? Is it really to be participatory?
2. How will decisions get made?
3. What are the research aims?
4. Who is the target population of interest?
5. How will the research be funded?
6. What will be our organization's and/or my role in the project?
7. Will the time be compensated?
8. Who will own the data? What will happen to the data in the future after the project is completed?
9. What benefits will the project leave behind in the community (skills, programming, policy, infrastructure, capacity building)?
10. What is the dissemination plan for this research?

Questions for community partners to ask themselves prior to engaging in CBPR

1. Does this study address an important problem relevant to my community and my constituents?
2. How does the research aim fit with the mission of my organization?
3. Do we have the capacity to participate? Space? Staff? Time?
4. What are our conflicting priorities?
5. What will be the impact of doing research on my organization's ability to get its core work accomplished?
6. Will the results lead to action that will help my community?

Questions for CBPR researchers to ask themselves prior to engaging in CBPR

1. Do I have connections in the community?
2. Do I know enough about the community, its makeup, assets, and challenges?
3. Do I have the time to invest in and develop relationships?
4. Do I have the support of a mentor who has experience in CBPR?
5. Do I possess cultural humility?

the organizational capacity to participate in the research project? Each of these issues can create problems if it is inadequately addressed beforehand.

Specific details for assessing readiness from the community perspective will be further discussed in Chapter 5.

❖ RULES OF PARTNERSHIP

Once a CBPR partnership is established, it is important that roles and responsibilities are outlined. By answering the questions posed for research readiness, partners can explore the details of who will do what, where, and when and mutually determine the organizational structure for the project itself. Some CBPR investigators and their community partners will choose to enter into more formal relationship in order to clarify roles and responsibilities. A memorandum of understanding, or MOU, can be used to outline the expectations. The development of an MOU will require consensus from the entire group. Examples of areas to be addressed in a MOU include the following:

- Overview of the project
- Description of each party's responsibilities
- Time frame
- Deliverables or milestones
- Budget
- Publication/dissemination requirements

This MOU can help both academic and community partners negotiate up front how the project will unfold and may help avoid future disagreement. With or without an MOU, it is important to have a transparent process in which these items are outlined early in the CBPR project. Baker and colleagues (1999) point to a set of principles that may be helpful in guiding effective academic/community partnerships that include mutual respect, trust, and honoring partners' agendas.[26] Each partnership may want to discuss its governance structure and decision-making strategies as part of this process. How will conflict be handled? What does each party hope to gain from the project and what are their plans for dissemination? In the Everett process, at the very beginning, the researcher said that one of her goals was to write an article for a peer-reviewed journal. She offered authorship to anyone in the group who was interested and discussed what would be expected of authors. Several community members said they wanted to be included, while others opted out. Similarly, the community partners wanted to host a large community forum to discuss the results of the research at the end of the project. There was money set aside for this activity in the budget, and a timeline was agreed upon in the CAB's first meeting. While this dual strategy does not always result in a smooth CBPR process, it can help avert pitfalls and satisfy the goals of both the academics and the community partners.

❖ MAINTAINING PARTNERSHIPS

As a CBPR partnership moves forward through a project, there will be an ongoing need to maintain transparency, communication, and engagement. New concerns will emerge from the community that will need to be addressed. The researcher will need to be fully prepared to listen to all the voices, and the partnership will need to navigate difficult decisions. However, with a strong foundation of mutual trust, these obstacles can be overcome and a fruitful relationship developed.

❖ CONCLUSION

In summary, community in CBPR can be defined in multiple ways. In general, it represents groups of people with shared concerns. As CBPR researchers define the community in which they intend to work, they need to learn about the strengths and assets of that community. This is a process that requires actively engaging with community members, learning about community norms, and visiting the community. As they begin to engage with community partners, they must understand the context in which these partners live their lives. The success or failure of a CBPR project rests on the strength of the academic/community partnership regardless of whether the community engages the researcher or the researcher seeks out community members.

❖ QUESTIONS AND ACTIVITIES

Activities

In the classroom: Have students map out a community as a group that they are familiar with, including its assets. Have them brainstorm strategies for getting to know the community, including suggestions about key stakeholders.

Out of the classroom: Have students take a tour of a local community, including institutions as well as important community landmarks (houses of worship, city hall, schools, parks, memorials). When they return, have the group discuss what their observations told them about the nature of the community (i.e., Were buildings in good repair? Were stores open? Were people walking about?).

Using a fishbowl exercise, have students role-play a first meeting between a researcher and a community partner while other students watch. The researcher's agenda is to find and seek out potential areas for research, while the community partner's agenda is to garner resources for her or his community program for youth development.

After the role play, have student observers describe what went well and what could improve in this relationship. Have students who participated in the role play describe their inner dialogue during the meeting.

1. What was the primary objective of the researcher? Was he or she able to establish a relationship with the community partner?

2. Were the agendas of researcher and community partner at odds? Compatible? Did they trust one another?

3. What challenges did you see in the interaction?

Questions for Discussion

1. What are some of the major strategies for getting to know a community of interest?

2. What might be the makeup of a community advisory board for a CBPR study on HIV/AIDs in an urban community. How might you go about convening such a group?

3. How do power dynamics influence in a CBPR project?

❖ NOTES

1.   MacQueen KM, McLellan E, Metzger DS, Kegeles S, Strauss RP, Scotti R, Blanchard L, Trotter RT. What is community? An evidence-based definition for participatory public health. *American Journal of Public Health*. 2001 Dec;91(12):1929–38.

2.   Jewkes R, Murcott A. Community representatives: representing the "community"? *Social Science & Medicine.* 1998 Apr;46(7):843–58.

3.   Hillery G. Definitions of community: areas of agreement. *Rural Sociology.* 1955;20:111–23.

4.   Mckeown TC, Rubinstein RA, Kelly JG. Anthropology, the meaning of community and prevention. In: Jason LA, Hess RE, Felner RD, Moritsugu JN, eds. *Prevention: Toward a Multidisciplinary Approach.* New York, NY: Haworth Press; 1987:35–64.

5.   Lee D, Newby H. *The Problem of Sociology: An Introduction to the Discipline.* London, England: Unwin Hyman Ltd.; 1983.

6.   Chavis DM, Newbrough J. The meaning of "community" in community psychology. *Journal of Community Psychology.* 1986 Oct;14(4):335–40.

7.   Patrick D, Wickizer T. Community and health. In: Amick B, Levine S, Tarlov A, Walsh DC, eds. *Society and Health.* New York, NY: Oxford University Press; 1995:4–92.

8.   Wellman B, Wortley S. Different strokes from different folks: community ties and social support. *American Journal of Sociology.* 1990 Nov;96(3): 558–88.

9.   McMillan DW, Chavis DM. Sense of community: a definition and theory. *American Journal of Community Psychology.* 1986 Jan;14(1):6–23.

10.   Hawe P. Capturing the meaning of "community" in community intervention evaluation: some contributions from community psychology. *Health Promotion International.* 1994;9(3):199–210.

11.   Sarason SB. *A Psychological Sense of Community. Prospects for a Community Psychology.* San Francisco, CA: Jossey Bass; 1974.

12.   Clinical and Translational Science Awards Consortium. Community Engagement Key Function Committee Task Force on the Principles of Community Engagement. *Principles of Community Engagement.* 2nd ed. Rockville, MD: NIH; 2011.

13.   Minkler M, Wallerstein N., eds. *Community-Based Participatory Research for Health.* San Francisco, CA: Jossey-Bass; 2003.

14.   Israel BA, Eng E, Schulz AJ, Parker EA, ed. *Methods in Community-Based Participatory Research for Health.* San Francisco, CA: Jossey-Bass; 2005.

15.   Israel BA, Lichtenstein R, Lantz P, McGranaghan R, Allen A, Guzman JR, Softley D, Maciak B. The Detroit Community-Academic Urban Research Center: development, implementation, and evaluation. *Journal of Public Health Management & Practice.* 2001 Sep;7(5):1–19.

16.   Taylor E, Marino D, Rasor-Greenhalgh S, Hudak S. Navigating practice and academic change in collaborative partnership with a community advisory board. *Journal of Allied Health.* 2010 Fall;39(3):e105–10.

17.   Silvestre AJ, Quinn SJ, Rinaldo CR. A twenty-two-year-old community advisory board: health research as an opportunity for social change. *Journal of Community Practice.* 2010 Jan 1;18(1):58–75.

18.   Blumenthal DS. A community coalition board creates a set of values for community-based research. *Preventing Chronic Disease: Public Health Research, Practice, and Policy.* 2006 January; 3(1):1–7.

19.   Health Safety Net-HSN (Free Care): an overview. MassResources.org; http://www.massresources.org/pages.cfm?contentID=50&pageID=13&Subpages=yes. Cited May 23, 2010.

20.   Hacker K, Chu J, Leung C, Marra R, Pirie A, Brahimi M, English M, Beckmann J, Acevedo-Garcia D, Marlin RP. The impact of Immigration and Customs Enforcement on immigrant health: perceptions of immigrants in Everett, Massachusetts, USA. *Social Science & Medicine.* 2011 Aug;73(4):586–94.

21.   Hacker K, Collins J, Gross-Young L, Almeida S, Burke N. Coping with youth suicide and overdose: one community's efforts to investigate, intervene, and prevent suicide contagion. *Crisis.* 2008;29(2):86–95.

22.   Taking It to the Curbside: Engaging Communities to Create Sustainable Change for Health. Conference, Boston, MA; 2010.

23.   Becker BA, Israel B, Allen AJ, III. Strategies and techniques for effective group process in CBPR partnerships. In: Israel BA, Eng E, Schulz A, Parker E, eds. *Methods in Community-Based Participatory Research for Health.* San Francisco, CA: Jossey-Bass; 2005;52.

24.   Chavez V, Duran B, Baker EA, Avila MM, Wallerstein N. The dance of race and privilege in CBPR. In: Minkler M, Wallerstein N, eds. *Community-Based Participatory Research for Health.* 2nd ed. San Francisco, CA: Jossey-Bass; 2008:91.

25.   Tervalon M, Murray-Garcia J. Cultural humility versus cultural competence: a critical distinction in defining physician training outcomes in multicultural education. *Journal of Health Care for the Poor and Underserved.* 1998 May;9(2):117–25.

26.   Baker EA, Homan S, Schonhoff R, Kreuter M. Principles of practice for academic/practice/community research partnerships. *American Journal of Preventive Medicine.*1999 Apr;16(3 Suppl):86–93.

3

Methods for CBPR

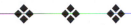

"Does CBPR add value to health research, or is the very premise of involving communities in the conduct of research contradictory to the tenets of 'science' defined traditionally as expert based and objective? Does CBPR truly shift the power relations between the observer and observed? And if so, does this serve the public health agenda of improving the science on which that agenda is based?"[1]

The engagement of community partners in the research enterprise is critical for improving human health and advancing science.[2] CBPR is an approach in which community members are actively involved in every facet of the research, shaping it, conducting it, interpreting results, and disseminating findings.[3] This approach not only changes traditional research paradigms but also has implications for the way we think about the scientific enterprise. When research is intimately connected to the communities under study, it should enhance the value of research for those communities. But will that mean that the results of the research can also be applied outside that community? As CBPR researchers, we must employ rigorous methods that approach the problem in a systematic way and have the potential for generalizability while also incorporating a participatory framework. Another way of thinking about the CBPR approach is that it requires research methods that simultaneously meet standards of scientific merit and acceptability and feasibility for community partners. To help the investigator better understand how methods are considered in CBPR, this chapter will describe:

1. Advantages and challenges of CBPR in the research process

2. The research question

3. Conceptual models and theorizing

4. Choice of methods

5. Sampling

6. Design considerations

❖ ADVANTAGES AND CHALLENGES OF
   CBPR IN THE RESEARCH PROCESS

The research process involves a series of steps that include theory, hypotheses, data collection, and analysis (see Figure 3.1).[4] Theory helps us make sense of interrelated phenomena in the social world.[4]

Figure 3.1   The Research Circle

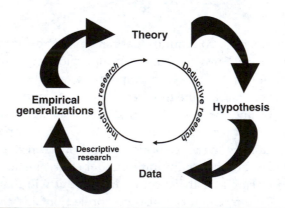

Source: Schutt, R. *Investigating the Social World* 6e, p. 42. Copyright © 2009 SAGE Publications.

Hypotheses are educated guesses about relationships between two or more characteristics that are usually based on observation or the literature. They can be proven true or false through the research process that includes data collection and analysis. While CBPR utilizes all the same steps as any research process, community participation creates an added layer that poses both challenges and opportunities for the research process. Perhaps one of the most important advantages of CBPR is its ability to enhance certain dimensions of validity and authenticity. CBPR offers an opportunity for colearning—that is, the researcher learns from the community as the community learns from the researcher.

In Schutt's book *Investigating the Social World*,[4] various facets of validity and authenticity are defined. *Validity* refers to how accurately your research conclusions correspond to the real world. The three dimensions of validity include measurement validity, generalizability, and causal validity. *Measurement validity* focuses on our ability to actually measure what we think we are measuring. *Generalizability* exists when our conclusions hold true for the community, population, or setting we specify. *Sample generalizability* refers to our ability to generalize from the sample to the population, while *external validity* or *cross-population validity* refers to our ability to generalize our findings from one group to other groups, populations, and settings. *Causal validity* refers to the state when your conclusion that A leads to B is correct.[4] The advantages and disadvantaged of achieving each form of validity in CBPR will be addressed throughout this chapter.

Finally, *authenticity* refers to how well the resulting understanding of the social process produced by the research reflects the various perspectives of participants in the setting.[4] The CBPR approach increases authenticity, as community participation assists with making the research more relevant to the community under study. This is one of the most unique and important aspects of CBPR. It offers the researcher a window into a perspective that he or she would normally find inaccessible. The colearning process inherent in CBPR enhances authenticity dramatically by providing insight into the research process from multiple perspectives. In our Everett, Massachusetts, example, where we studied the implications of Immigration and Customs Enforcement (ICE) on immigrant health, the advantages of the CBPR process included the provision of a timely topic area that was particularly important to the community—ICE and immigrant health—along with important input from the immigrant communities. Neither of these would have been identified without the participation of community members.

The process of coeducating and colearning that occurs in CBPR has the advantage of providing a multidisciplinary approach to problem solving. Not only are there opportunities for sharing information and knowledge across the community/academic continuum, but there is joint learning that occurs throughout the experience that has implications for future action, sustainability, and research. If the researcher is open to the ways the community might answer pressing questions, it can result in better, more applicable approaches to generating knowledge.

But CBPR also poses methodological challenges. With increased relevancy, there may be questions about validity and external generalizability, since the work is locally based. There may also be challenges to design and methods. Community participation may influence choice of the research questions, sampling methods, and the recruitment of the sample. The preferred methods of community partners may conflict with those of researchers. In this chapter, we will discuss important elements of the research process and the unique methodological advantages and challenges of CBPR.

❖ THE RESEARCH QUESTION

Working with community partners to hone a research question can be an invigorating and creative experience. Their insights, provided from multiple perspectives, can reveal aspects of the problem that the researcher may never have considered. However, a community's questions may not always reflect what social scientists have identified as the key unanswered questions. In general, community partners often have broad questions that reflect current problems in their community, and their knowledge of existing literature may be lacking. They want to understand youth violence or underperforming students or reasons for homelessness. In response, it is necessary to refine the questions such that the researcher may need to broaden his or her questions and the community may need to narrow theirs. In Everett, Massachusetts, the community had a particular concern: they were worried that immigrants in their community were experiencing health problems due to immigration enforcement. When they approached the researcher, they had a broad question that they wanted to explore: Does ICE impact immigrant health? The refinement process was collaborative and multifaceted. First, the researchers provided a review and interpretation of the existing literature on the topic in the initial meetings of the academic/community research team. Community partners may or may not be aware of the literature on a topic. They are unlikely to be familiar with academic articles or possess knowledge to interpret them. Yet understanding the state of the research and the new and emerging questions is an important task in the research process. This is one of the skill sets that the researcher brings to the CBPR process. For Everett partners, the literature revealed that little work had been done in this area. The limited prior literature was focused on experiences with a previously repealed California law that limited immigrants' access to health care. The literature review helped to identify a host of new questions that the community/research partnership reviewed and considered. In addition, the team was able to establish the need for this work at both the local and national levels. Questions that emerged from the literature included: Does immigration enforcement lead to lower use of health services? Does fear of deportation result in worsening of health conditions? Does deportation fear differ across immigrant groups?

In order to effectively work through the development and refinement of the research questions in CBPR, both researchers and community partners need to be able to get their perspectives heard and incorporated. Question refinement and hypothesis generation can take some time but will have a secondary effect of deepening collaboration. In addition, the conceptual framework can help the CAB identify effective methods and short- and long-term outcomes.

❖ CONCEPTUAL MODEL AND THEORIZING

A conceptual model or framework provides a visual representation of how a set of factors relate to one another and are thought to impact or lead to a target outcome. It can be extremely helpful in connecting the research questions to theory and further refining the hypotheses. As a next step, researchers in Everett took the information gleaned from the literature along with perceptions of community members and drafted a conceptual model of the project. Building a conceptual model was an excellent tool to help the partners identify the mechanism by which they believed that ICE was having an impact on immigrant health. In turn, this model helped the research team further develop research questions and hypotheses. In addition to the conceptual model, the researchers provided information on social theories. In particular for this project, theories of social capital and segmented assimilation theories were presented.[5-7] Using the draft conceptual model as a starting point, the team had an opportunity to provide input on the mechanism behind the impact of ICE on immigrant health. This exercise helped the community build its theory about the elements of the problem it was exploring.

To demonstrate one of the values of CBPR, the two versions of the conceptual framework are shown below. The version initially presented by researchers changed substantially as community members provided their contributions. While researchers thought about the implications of increased fear on individual mental health and stress levels (Figure 3.2), community members pointed out that much of the problem was being driven by having or not having a driver's license. Immigrants who did not have driver's licenses were at risk for being

Figure 3.2   Conceptual Framework for the Impact of ICE Efforts on Immigrant Health

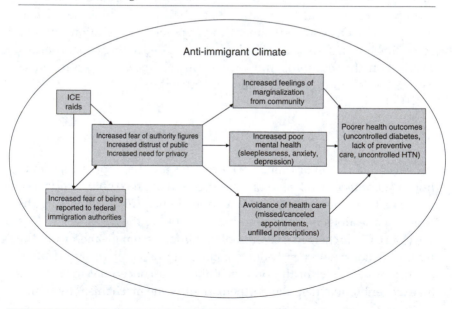

Source: Reproduced by permission from the Institute for Community Health, Cambridge, MA; 2011.

arrested by police when they were stopped for even a minor traffic violation. If arrested, fingerprinting created high anxiety, as immigrants feared their information would be shared with immigration authorities. This was incorporated into a final conceptual framework for the project (Figure 3.3).

The visual aid along with the literature review previously mentioned helped the group further refine its set of research questions and associated hypotheses. In CBPR, once the research process begins, new and emerging research questions will surface, as the process is iterative and tends to move from broad to more specific. Here are some examples of research questions that were informed by the literature review, the conceptual framework, and theory:

1. What were the perceptions of different immigrant communities about local police and the relationship to ICE?

    Hypothesis 1: Immigrants did not distinguish between law enforcement and ICE.

Figure 3.3   Conceptual Framework for the Impact of ICE Efforts on Immigrant Health (Version 2)

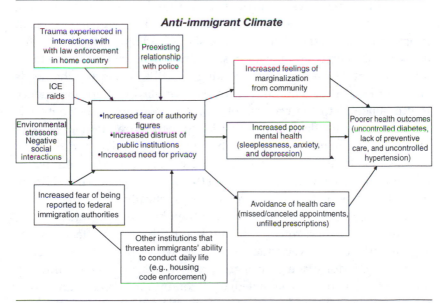

Source: Reprinted from *Social Science and Medicine 73* (2011) 586–594; Hacker, K., Chu, J., Leung, C., Marra, R., Pirie, A., Brahimi, M., English, M., Beckmann, J., Acevedo-Garcia, D., & Marlin, R. "The impact of Immigration and Customs Enforcement on immigrant health: Perceptions of immigrants in Everett, Massachusetts, USA" page 588. Copyright 2011 with permission from Elsevier.

Hypothesis 2: Undocumented immigrants were more likely to have their health more negatively impacted by ICE than those that were documented.

2. How did the presence of ICE in the community impact access to health care?

Hypothesis: People exposed to high rates of deportation in their community were afraid to go out of their houses and would therefore miss doctors' appointments.

3. How did immigrants who came from countries where they had experienced trauma differ from immigrants who did not experience trauma in their response to ICE?

Hypothesis: Immigrants from countries where they had experienced trauma would be more likely to have physical symptoms of stress resulting from ICE compared to those who did not experience trauma.

❖ CHOICE OF METHODS

Once the research question is defined and the hypotheses delineated, it is time to match the methods to the question(s). As with any research project, the methods used in CBPR should adequately address the question of interest and meet the standards of rigor used in scientific investigation. However, when working in CBPR, balancing the needs and desires of the community with the standard of rigorous science is fundamental to the premise of CBPR. The community context is fluid and requires flexibility not typically seen in traditional research. Decisions about methods should be made jointly. The acceptability of those methods—that is, whether the community considers methods appropriate for its context—must also be assessed. In addition, feasibility, or whether the research can practically be carried out in the community, will need to be determined by the community. Thus, determining the best research methods for the project often requires a give and take between the researcher, who possesses knowledge of scientific inquiry and its design and methods, and the community members, who possess knowledge of community context and what is possible for political, historical, and practical reasons. With the help of community partners, novel and more applicable methods may be identified that provide more appropriate strategies for generating knowledge than those proposed by the researcher.

A discussion of the limitations and strengths of particular methods should be a group process. There are some pivotal research concepts that can facilitate the discussion, particularly the concept and dimensions of validity and systematic bias. Community members are often unfamiliar with these terms, and it is contingent upon researchers to translate them to their community partners. These concepts are critical for understanding the strengths and limitations of the chosen research methods and the impact on conclusions. The resulting strength of evidence will be dependent on eliminating as much systematic bias as possible and maximizing validity. These fundamental research concepts can help community partners understand the rationale for certain methods, what is involved in increasing research rigor (Figure 3.4), and more importantly, what conclusions they will be able to draw based on the chosen methods and design.

To date, it is still rare for CBPR to utilize experimental designs,[3] which limits the extent to which CBPR can establish causal validity. Experimental designs require at least one group that receives some treatment and a control or comparison group that does not receive the treatment. Participants are randomly assigned to the control group. Random sampling is a sampling method that identifies subjects through chance. It can help to decrease sampling bias, which is the "over or underrepresentation of some population characteristics in a sample due to the method used to select the sample."[4] True experimental design is often not feasible in community settings for reasons

Figure 3.4   Increasing Research Rigor

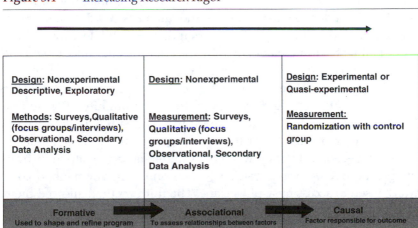

Source: Reproduced by permission from the Institute for Community Health, Cambridge, MA; 2011.

that will be discussed later. In addition, the need for highly controlled methods may not be readily accepted by community partners or necessary to answer the question under study. Today, it is much more common to see nonexperimental methods utilized in CBPR studies.

Nonexperimental Methods

Nonexperimental methods include qualitative methods such as focus groups and interviews and quantitative methods such as retrospective data review and surveys. These methods have the advantage of being easily adapted to a participatory approach. With training, community partners can be involved in conducting observations, taking notes, facilitating focus groups, or developing and conducting surveys. They can also be involved in the recruitment of participants for any of these activities. Each of these methods also has potential utility for their future work, thus building important community capacity. For example, community partners may utilize surveys as part of community needs assessment and evaluation activities.

In our Everett example, community members wanted to learn more from those most affected by the issue under study. Given the subject, formative and associational methods that would test the hypotheses were chosen. From the onset, the research team was aware that the results of their work were likely to be limited to Everett and not have cross-population generalizability. However, since little had been published on the subject, they also felt they would be adding to the literature on the topic. The team agreed on a combination of methods that included both qualitative and quantitative data collection. These included (1) focus groups, (2) a survey, and (3) interviews. These would allow for triangulation of data in order to better understand the situation and plan for future interventions.

The partners chose to conduct a series of focus groups with the five dominant language groups in their community: Portuguese (Brazilian), Spanish (Central American), Haitian (Creole), Arabic (Moroccan), and English (for those immigrants that were bilingual in English). Secondarily, they wanted to understand the situation from the perspective of local physicians, so an online survey methodology was chosen to access busy physicians. The third method allowed them to learn more about the problem from key community stakeholders through a series of hour-long interviews.[8] These three methods all lent themselves to a collaborative, participatory approach.

Focus groups are designed to get the opinion of a group.[4] To begin, Everett team members identified the key questions they felt were important and developed and piloted the moderator's guide. The moderator's guide included a range of questions that were designed to test the hypotheses previously identified. For example, there was a series of questions that asked about relationships with local law enforcement to try to tease out how immigrants felt about police and whether they associated them with ICE. Once the guide was completed, the group decided to have community partners facilitate the focus groups in the appropriate languages. Toward this goal, the researchers trained the community leaders to facilitate the focus groups and serve as note takers. Community partners also had the ability to recruit focus group participants. Through participants contacting other potential participants, more than 50 people were recruited to participate. Focus groups were held in community settings to minimize anxiety of participants.[8]

The second method that Everett partners selected was an online survey for community health providers in order to determine whether these providers were identifying an impact on their immigrant patients. Since there were no available surveys that had been previously validated, the team developed its own questions. While CBPR allows for the mutual development of community-relevant questions, this may sacrifice measurement validity—that is, ensuring that "a measure measures what we think it measures."[4] These community-developed questions have not been field tested, nor have they gone through validity testing. This is not an uncommon situation in CBPR. While community partners provide excellent ideas for question development, they generally do not have extensive experience writing effective survey questions, which may lead to confusing phrasing, problems with response categories, overlapping dimensions of concepts, and other survey errors. Researchers can help their community partners with survey design and improve measurement validity by building on existing instruments and refining and testing questions before release. The benefit of survey methods along with the insight of community partners can work together to produce high-quality survey instruments.

Evaluation Research

Another design strategy that is frequently seen in CBPR is the use of evaluation research to gauge the impact of particular interventions or assess the needs of the community. Today, the incorporation of evaluative methods in community health programming is widespread. Since the 1990s, more and more grant-funded programs require some level of evaluation, that is, "Show us how you intend to measure the outcomes of your proposed program." Whether it is a new or existing intervention, community members are often very interested in determining what programs and services work or might not work in their communities. Evaluation research is generally considered the "systematic collection of information about the activities, characteristics, and outcomes of programs."[2] This might include needs assessment and formative research as well as experimental intervention research. Much of what is done in CBPR could fall within the definition of evaluation research. When evaluation researchers focus on the identification of the effects of a program, they frequently utilize a pre-post design with or without a control group. This type of design can be represented with a logic model, which is a descriptive model of how a program operates.[4] Using a logic model with community partners can also be a helpful exercise, particularly if doing intervention research. The logic model has been used by program developers and evaluators to map out the premise behind the program and identify the measurable indicators for evaluation.[9] A template for logic models is included in Figure 3.5.

Figure 3.5   How to Read a Logic Model

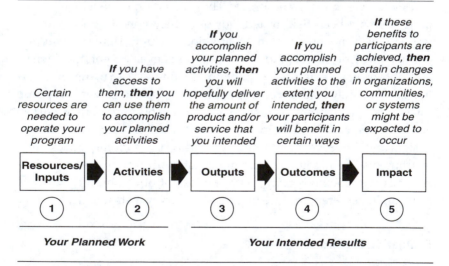

Source: W.K. Kellogg Foundation Logic Model Development Guide, W.K. Kellogg Foundation Battlecreek MI Jan 2004 Item #1209 p.3 Available online http://www.wkkf.org/knowledge-center/resources/2006/02/ WK-Kellogg-Foundation-Logic-Model-Development-Guide.aspx

Many community members will benefit from learning basic evaluation techniques and incorporating appropriate measures into their work for process improvement. This process improvement in community programming resembles the Plan Do Study Act process used throughout industry. Figure 3.6, shown previously in Chapter 1, demonstrates how research can be used for process improvement. Community partners learn to question, study, and assess their results and then adapt and adjust for improvement. An academic partner can assist communities with the development of a logic model, framing of achievable short- and long-term goals, and identification of measures and measurement tools, as well as choice of evaluation design.

Overall, the research design for any CBPR project should be appropriate to answer the question posed. In our Everett example, some important points were identified. First, the background literature provided by the researcher helped inform the community about existing evidence in the area. Second, the joint effort to build a conceptual framework provided a starting point for determining the appropriate methods for the project. The process also allowed researchers to better understand the current community political and cultural context and

Figure 3.6   Research for Process Improvement

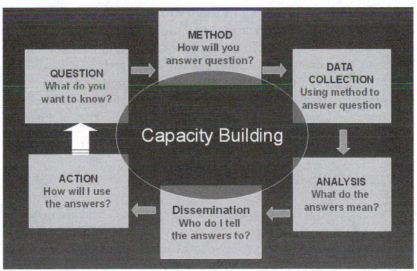

Source: Reproduced by permission from the Institute for Community Health, Cambridge, MA; 2011.

revealed previously unknown factors that might influence immigrants' response to ICE.

❖ SAMPLING

The concept of sampling is of major import in the research process, yet it can be difficult to explain and manage in CBPR. Appropriate sampling will help minimize sampling bias—that is, when characteristics of the sample do not correlate to those of the population from which the sample is drawn. While one of the benefits of CBPR is that community partners can reach out to the community and thus improve recruitment success and hopefully sample generalizability, they may not consider the importance of keeping track of who refuses participation or exactly how many people they approach. Yet if they do not understand the concept of sampling bias, they may end up recruiting a group of people that does not reflect the characteristics of the population of interest and negates the validity of their work by drawing inaccurate conclusions based on problematic data. Therefore, just as it is important for community partners to explain the nuances of outreach and engagement to researchers, it is important for researchers to assist community partners in understanding the value of sample generalizability so that critical mistakes can be avoided. In Everett, community partners were so enthusiastic about conducting focus groups, they did not initially think about documenting their recruitment process. Part of the researcher's responsibility is to help build capacity for research in their community partners. A researcher can explain important research concepts such as selection bias, validity, and sampling. When partners understand why it is important to collect this data in a specific manner, they are more apt to comply, and over time, these concepts will become part of the CBPR process as partners incorporate their meaning and value.

❖ DESIGN CONSIDERATIONS

Community and academic incentives to engage in CBPR are generally different. Communities are likely to be more interested in the results of research activities as they pertain to local action rather than their implications for the field. Their time frames for action may be shorter and their tolerance lower for tightly controlled studies. This is one of the fundamental challenges in CBPR: How can research be meaningful to the community while also providing cross-population generalizability outside the community? To some extent, the answer to this question lies in whether the population under study and the community context itself was comparable to other populations in other communities. While experimental designs will help achieve cross-population generalizability of study findings, they are not the only factor to be considered. Today, CBPR researchers are attempting to better understand these contextual factors inherent in communities and CBPR partnerships that shape the "nature of the research and the partnership"[10] and ultimately help disseminate effective approaches.

While the number of experimental trials conducted using CBPR is increasing, to date, the majority of CBPR studies have largely been observational and quasi-experimental (studies that do not randomly assign participants but use matched control groups instead).[3, 11] As noted in the Agency for Healthcare Research and Quality (AHRQ) review of 2004,[3] CBPR builds trust with communities and improves relevancy and recruitment, but the scientific rigor of CBPR is still in question. One reason for this conclusion is the lack of experimental methods that pose threats to causal validity. Why is it challenging to use randomization in CBPR? In part, community partners may be hesitant to consider randomization, which excludes some community members from the receipt of an intervention while offering it to others. They may feel that restricting service is inappropriate, especially for disadvantaged populations. For example, a behavioral intervention that provides education and peer support to help teen mothers practice safe sex should be offered to all regardless of whether the program is ultimately shown to "work." The community may place more value on obtaining additional services than on testing the value of those services. This may be frustrating to the researcher who wants to identify scientific evidence for the uptake of new community interventions.

Another consideration is the feasibility of conducting a randomized experimental design in a community setting. The CBPR partnership needs to assess whether this level of experimental research can actually be achieved. These studies generally require more time and resources than other designs and are most often led by the researcher. They may not lend themselves to a participatory approach. Most importantly, they require extensive control over all elements of the study. Thus, undertaking a randomized experimental design using a CBPR approach will require the partnership to negotiate roles and responsibilities, especially since the flexibility inherent in a CBPR approach may directly conflict with the control needed to conduct the research. Rather than individual randomization, strategies such as cluster randomization, in which clusters of social groups are randomized (churches, community clinics, schools), or delayed interventions, in which the comparison group becomes the experimental group and receives the intervention in a delayed fashion, may be more palatable for community partners.

While the challenges are numerous, experimental designs are possible. As CBPR partnerships evolve, they may be more likely to consider a higher level of rigor in their research methodology based on their trust of the researcher and their understanding of the value of experimental research designs. This may follow from earlier pilot work in which lessons have been learned.

❖ CONCLUSION

Refining the research question is an important place to start in CBPR. Once achieved, developing a consensus around methods that are rigorous and simultaneously feasible and acceptable to community partners is critical. The researcher who understands the inherent limitations of certain methods will not only achieve better long-term results but also is more likely to build community partnerships that endure for the future.

As partnerships mature and community partners gain confidence with research methods, more complex designs may be possible. Throughout the research process, there is an ongoing colearning process that is unique to a CBPR approach. Both researchers and community partners build their capacity, and as partnerships deepen and endure, the possibilities for future beneficial CBPR projects increase.

❖ QUESTIONS AND ACTIVITIES

Activities

Have students discuss the steps to the research process as they differ in CBPR compared to traditional research.

1. Consider the following case:

Community members want to address violence in their community. They want to understand why young people in one area of the city are involved in the majority of the drive-by shootings. They ask you as a researcher to help them learn about the risk factors for violence in youth.

Describe the process for refining the research question in a way that utilizes the principles of CBPR.

2. A community group is interested in trying to identify whether a program for overweight children can actually impact BMI. The program is a 10-week educational intervention delivered at a community youth development site by youth leaders.

Using this case study, have students map out a logic model of the program and include appropriate measures.

3. You are approached by a community partner that runs a program for out-of-school youth designed to help them get their high school certificates. The program does not seem to be having the desired impact. The program runs for six sessions. Staff currently keep records of participation and high school completion.

Describe how you would approach the evaluation of this project and the methods you might suggest. Discuss the relative merits of an experimental versus nonexperimental design within the context of CBPR.

Questions

1. Discuss the three dimensions of validity and give examples of how a CBPR project might strengthen or inhibit the successful achievement of these dimensions.

2. Describe the challenges in conducting a randomized experiment using CBPR. What would be the concerns of the community? Are there other strategies for randomization that might be more acceptable to community partners? Describe them.

3. What are some strategies for discussing the advantages of more rigorous designs with community partners?

4. How can you as a researcher assist your community partners in understanding the evidence base related to a question of interest?

❖ NOTES

1. Minkler M, Wallerstein N., eds. *Comunity-Based Participatory Research for Health.* San Francisco, CA: Jossey-Bass; 2003:241.

2. Clinical and Translational Science Awards Consortium. Community Engagement Key Function Committee Task Force on the Principles of Community Engagement. *Principles of Community Engagement.* 2nd ed. Rockville, MD: NIH; 2011.

3. Viswanathan M, Ammerman A, Eng E, Gartlehner G, Lohr KN, Griffith D, Rhodes S, Samuel-Hodge C, Maty S, Lux, L, Webb L, Sutton SF, Swinson T, Jackman A, Whitener L. *Community-Based Participatory Research: Assessing the Evidence.* Evidence Report/Technology Assessment No. 99 (Prepared by RTI–University of North Carolina Evidence-based Practice Center). AHRQ Publication 04-E022-2. Rockville, MD: Agency for Healthcare Research and Quality. July 2004.

4. Schutt RK. *Investigating the Social World.* 6th ed. Thousand Oaks, California: Pine Forge Press; 2009:38, 42, 51–53, 158, 345, 50, 411.

5. Kawachi I, Subramanian SV, Almeida-Filho N. A glossary for health inequalities. *Journal of Epidemiology and Community Health.* 2002 Sep;56(9):647–52.

6. Kim D, Subramanian SV, Kawachi I. Bonding versus bridging social capital and their associations with self rated health: a multilevel analysis of 40 US communities. *Journal of Epidemiology and Community Health.* 2006 Feb;60(2):116–22.

7. Portes A, Fernandez-Kelly P, Haller W. Segmented assimilation on the ground: the new second generation in early adulthood. *Ethnic and Racial Studies.* 2005 Nov;28(6):1000–40.

8. Hacker K, Chu J, Leung C, Marra R, Pirie A, Brahimi M, English M, Beckmann J, Acevedo-Garcia D, Marlin RP. The impact of Immigration and Customs Enforcement on immigrant health: perceptions of immigrants in Everett, Massachusetts, USA. *Social Science & Medicine.* 2011 Aug;73(4):586–94.

9. McLaughlin JA, Jordan GB. Logic models: a tool for telling your program's performance story. *Evaluation and Planning.* 1999 Spring;22(1):65–72.

10. Wallerstein N, Duran B. Community-based participatory research contributions to intervention research: the intersection of science and practice

to improve health equity. *American Journal of Public Health.* 2010 Apr 1;100 (Suppl 1):S40–46.

11.   De Las Nueces D, Hacker K, Digirolamo A, Hicks LS. A systematic review of community-based participatory research to enhance clinical trials in racial and ethnic minority groups. *Health Services Research.* 2012 Jun;47 (3 pt 2):1363–86.

Appendix of Key Terms[4]

Taken from R. K. Schutt, *Investigating the Social World.*

Theory
A logically interrelated set of propositions about empirical reality (p. 38)

Hypothesis
A tentative statement about empirical reality, involving a relationship between two or more variables (p. 42)

Variable
A characteristic or property that can vary (take on different values or attributes) (p. 42)

Validity
The state that exists when statements or conclusions about empirical reality are correct (p. 50)

Measurement validity
Exists when a measure measures what we think it measures (p. 50)

Generalizability
Exists when a conclusion holds true for the population, group, setting, or event that we say it does, given the conditions that we specify (p. 50)

Sample generalizability
Refers to the ability to generalize from a sample, or subset, of a larger population to that population itself (p. 51)

Cross-population generalizability (external validity)
Refers to the ability to generalize from findings about one group, population, or setting to other groups, populations, or settings (p. 51)

Causal validity
Exists when a conclusion that A leads to our results in B is correct (p. 50)

Authenticity
When the understanding of a social process or social setting is one that reflects fairly the various perspectives of participants in that setting (p. 50)

Sample
A subset of a population that is used to study the population as a whole (p. 149)

Program theory
A descriptive or prescriptive model of how a program operates and produces effects (p. 411)

Random sampling
A method of sampling that relies on a random, or chance, selection method so that every element of the sampling frame has a known probability of being selected (p. 157)

Systematic bias
Overrepresentation or underrepresentation of some population characteristics in a sample due to the method used to select the sample (p. 158)

Control group
A comparison group that receives no treatment (p. 223)

Quantitative methods
Methods such as surveys and experiments that record variation in social life in terms of quantities (p. 17)

Qualitative methods
Methods such as participant observation, intensive interviewing, and focus groups that are designed to capture social life as participants experience it rather than in categories predetermined by the researcher (p. 17)

Evaluation research

Research that describes or identifies the impact of social policies and programs (p. 395)

Selection bias

When characteristics of the experimental and comparison groups differ or when the group under study has some characteristics that biases their responses (in surveys or focus groups) (p. 238)

4

CBPR—Step by Step

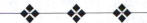

Now that you have an understanding of the underpinnings of CBPR, it is valuable to walk step by step through a project in order to understand the approach. As discussed in prior chapters, the fundamental steps in CBPR revolve around some salient concepts: community assessment, strategic goal setting, identification of problems, formulating research design, research conduct, analysis/interpretation, and dissemination, including action. In this chapter, we will present "How to do CBPR" utilizing case examples and walking the reader through the various stages of a CBPR project.

1. First stage: Defining the community, engaging the community, community needs assessment, identifying the research question

2. Second stage: Design/hypothesis testing, roles and responsibilities in the conduct of the research

3. Third stage: Analysis, interpretation and results, dissemination and action

The first case example is from Everett, Massachusetts, where a CBPR study of the impact of Immigration and Customs Enforcement on immigrant health occurred in 2010. The second case is from Cambridge, Massachusetts, where a CBPR project examined weight disparities among the African American population. The third case example is from a suicide cluster investigation in Somerville, Massachusetts, from 2002 to 2006. All three cases were presented in Chapter 1 and are presented here again for the reader's convenience.

Example 1. Immigrant Health in Everett, Massachusetts

Picture 4.1   Everett Community Partners

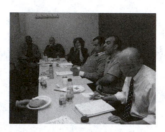

Source: Reproduced by permission from the Institute for Community Health, Cambridge, MA; 2011.

As described in Chapter 1, Everett, Massachusetts, has seen an influx of immigrants coming from countries such as Brazil, Haiti, Guatemala, and Morocco. Everett is a small city of about 37,000 with reasonable rents and proximity to Boston. While there have been tensions in the community about issues related to immigration, such as housing and parking, it is only recently that the increased activity of Immigration and Customs Enforcement (ICE) has created challenges for the immigrant community. In particular, with increases in deportation and detention, immigrants fear that they will be picked up by authorities and deported. Stories of immigrants missing health appointments because ICE was in the vicinity or having stress-related conditions such as sleeplessness, headaches, and weight loss were common. These concerns were raised by several of the immigrant advocacy groups and Everett community leaders, who felt that getting concrete information about this issue would facilitate changes in local policy. So they approached a familiar academic partner to join them in an investigation of the problem. Their goal was to learn more about the issue and then solve the problem and develop policy or programmatic interventions that would alleviate some of the stress that immigrants were experiencing.[1]

In this scenario, members of the target community approached the researcher to assist in answering what they saw as a pressing health and social issue in their community. While this may be perceived as a preferable CBPR initiator, there are many cases of CBPR researchers approaching a community with a research topic, particularly when they are familiar with members of that community.

Example 2: BMI Disparities in Cambridge, Massachusetts

Figure 4.1   The Cambridge H.E.L.P. Project

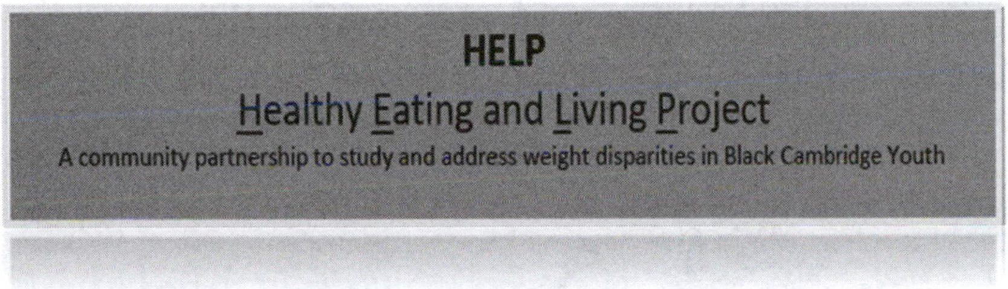

HELP

Healthy **E**ating and **L**iving **P**roject

A community partnership to study and address weight disparities in Black Cambridge Youth

Source: Reproduced by permission from the Institute for Community Health, Cambridge, MA; 2011.

Our second case as previously described, took place in Cambridge, Massachusetts over a 10-year period, schools, public health agencies, and researchers had combined forces to track childhood indicators of obesity. Annual height and weight measurements of children were taken by school personnel and provided to parents each year in the form of a healthy weight progress report.[2] Data accumulated through this process were available and allowed researchers to examine trends in childhood obesity as well as disparities among racial/ethnic groups.[3] The researcher noted that despite downward trends in BMI in the population overall, there were persistent and glaring disparities by race/ethnicity, with both Blacks and Hispanics carrying an undue burden of obesity. The researcher and a community colleague with whom she already had a relationship joined forces to pursue this line of inquiry. They started by discussing their concerns with several African American colleagues who were leaders in the community and were eager to work with them. Together, they approached other key leaders in the community, including a principal of a school with a large Black population. After exploring the existing data, they obtained a small amount of pilot funding to conduct several key stakeholder interviews with "positive deviants"—local African Americans who had made significant lifestyle changes and who had made progress toward attaining healthy weight. Using the results of these interviews, they applied for a larger pilot grant to conduct further analysis of existing data, collect more qualitative, contextual data, and to work with community partners to build appropriate interventions.

Example 3: Suicide Cluster in Somerville, Massachusetts: Real-Time Health Crisis

Figure 4.2   Suicide Attempts and Completed Suicides Among Somerville Residents Ages 10 to 24 Years

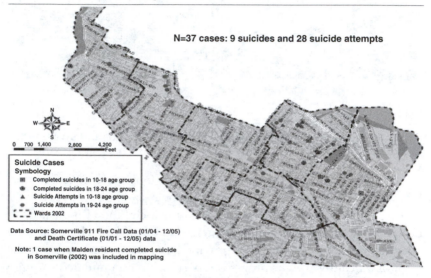

N=37 cases: 9 suicides and 28 suicide attempts

0   700 1,400   2,800   4,200 Feet

Suicide Cases Symbology
- Completed suicides in 10-18 age group
- Completed suicides in 18-24 age group
- Suicide Attempts in 10-18 age group
- Suicide Attempts in 19-24 age group
- Wards 2002

Data Source: Somerville 911 Fire Call Data (01/04 - 12/05) and Death Certificate (01/01 - 12/05) data

Note: 1 case when Malden resident completed suicide in Somerville (2002) was included in mapping

Source: Reproduced by permission from *Crisis*; Vol. 29(2): 86–95. © 2008 Hogrefe & Huber Publishers, www.hogrefe.com

As previously presented in Chapter 1, our third case took place in Somerville, Massachusetts, an urban city of 70,000 people that borders Cambridge, Massachusetts. Historically, Somerville has been home to working-class populations and in recent years, between gentrification and new immigration, the city's demography has changed substantially. Somerville has also been affected by long-term substance abuse problems, especially heroin and alcohol. In 2001, a young person took his own life, and this was followed soon after by oxycodone overdoses of two high school students. A local researcher with an interest and experience in adolescent suicide was concerned that this might represent the beginning of a suicide cluster. She had prior relationships with community partners and so approached the Health Department director and mayor to discuss her concerns and interest.

Loss of youth life to suicide and overdose sends enormous ripples of concern through any community, and in Somerville, the Health and School Departments examined data from their biannual teen health survey to determine if suicidal behaviors had changed. The teen survey noted that 21% of the students had seriously considered suicide, and 14% had attempted suicide during the last 12 months. This was substantially elevated over previous years and higher than the average for the state overall.

In order to respond to the situation and investigate further, the mayor convened several task forces and asked the researcher to join with community members and colead one of the task forces along with the Health Department Director. Other members included representation from the schools, the police, and community members, as well as additional experts in suicide clusters. The question posed by the community to the researcher was "How do we stop the youth suicide?" The researcher helped to reframe the question into two fundamental questions:

- Was this suicide and overdose activity significantly elevated from baseline?
- Were there common links between victims and was this a contagion/cluster?[2]

❖ FIRST STAGE: DEFINING THE COMMUNITY, ENGAGING THE COMMUNITY, COMMUNITY NEEDS ASSESSMENT, IDENTIFYING THE RESEARCH QUESTION

Each case presents a slightly different way to consider defining community. As an investigator, you need to consider what community you want to approach; this may have to do with your content area or with your current locale. Either way, you need to be aware of the boundaries around the community that you want to engage before taking your next steps. Community can be defined by geography, by condition, or by other common concerns/characteristics. If you want to work with immigrants, think through the groups that might represent this population and contact them. If you want to work with a geographic community, consider the organizations or institutions that serve the community. In the Everett case, the community essentially defined itself, and community members with a particular concern approached a familiar researcher. The group of people representing the immigrant community and those that provided services to them included a broad representation of the leaders from immigrant groups and local institutions, including schools, city government, and police. This self-defined community, however, did not fully represent the population of interest, and as the work proceeded, the researcher and the community members made efforts to expand their group to include more members from the target population: immigrant residents of Everett. Through community partners' social networks, introductions were made, and new members joined the CBPR project.

In contrast to this approach, it is not unusual for a researcher who is interested in exploring a specific topic to approach community partners. The challenge is whether the researcher's area of interest is also of interest to the community at large. If the researcher has done an adequate job of assessing the needs of a given community, this should not pose a problem. In the Cambridge case, it was the researcher who approached the African American community leaders in Cambridge, but several important points should be noted. First, the project was built on prior existing and trusting relationships. Thus, the researcher had excellent knowledge of the key stakeholders from the Black community. These stakeholders were well connected and had the potential to open doors to other community members to further the work. Second, the topic chosen for study expanded prior work that was already deemed to be of interest to this community—namely, despite increased community activities for healthy eating and active living, Black youth were still twice as likely to be overweight or obese compared to their White peers. The practice of CBPR is best built on mutual interest and existing relationships, as illustrated here. The researcher who has not done her or his homework to understand the issues facing the community will find CBPR more challenging and is less likely to be successful in such a pursuit.

In the Somerville example, the community was defined geographically, and the researcher and the community both identified the problem as it was occurring. The researcher pointed out the emerging problem to local leaders, including the mayor. Then, as the community began to coalesce around the issue, the researcher was brought in as a pivotal addition to the community task force and was able to add expertise. It was during the crisis that the researcher and community partners built new relationships and developed others. In this case, the researcher was really in the thick of the situation and acted as both a community partner and an investigator toward trying to find solutions.

In all three of these cases, it is hard to separate the "defining the community stage" from the "engagement stage." The very process of defining the community leads the researcher to develop relationships, walk the streets, learn the culture, and immerse him- or herself in the community of interest.

Steps 1 and 2: Defining and Engaging the Community and Community Needs Assessment

Once you have determined your target community, you will need to begin the engagement process. Start by examining any data available on the community of interest, then contact the local service and civic organizations and ask for an informational meeting, explore their websites, and learn what they provide. Census data are an excellent source when thinking about geographic populations. This information is available on the Census website[3] and can provide information on economic conditions as well as demography. In addition, local newspapers are helpful in learning about local politics. For specific populations, there are likely to be other sources available: immigrant advocacy groups, national associations, prior publications, and the like. Educating yourself about the community of interest before you try to engage its members will be helpful in your approach. In addition, in CBPR, don't go into your community engagement process with the particular research agenda in mind. You will need to better understand the community concerns before you can really focus on a particular research question. Otherwise, there is a chance your interest will not be of interest to your community partners, and you will find the mismatch of priorities frustrating.

How can one learn about current community concerns? In general, as noted above, existing data on community health and social issues are available through local sources such as school department reports, public health assessments, or statewide information on localities. In our Everett project, learning about Everett through its citywide website gave us information on the current issues and community resources. In addition, state data on health issues were available through the

Massachusetts Department of Public Health. These high-level data are helpful as you develop an understanding of the community, but nothing can replace showing up in the community and getting to know the local culture and important leaders. This is also the best strategy with which to begin your community engagement activities. Start with a basic needs assessment. Contact leaders of active community groups such as schools, community-based organizations, advocacy groups, religious groups, and service agencies. Meet with the directors and find out what they perceive as the challenges in their community. Think about where the likely places are that serve the population you are interested in studying. For example, if you are interested in maternal infant health, try working with local pediatricians or preschool programs. If you are interested in the elderly, contact senior centers. If you are interested in substance abuse, learn about the local substance abuse provider agencies. Visit the programs and meet their directors. Ask questions like: What was the stimulus for starting your organization? What do you see as the major issues facing your community? This process may seem onerous, but the results will provide an important foundation for future work. These early introductions will serve as the foundations of partnership as you and your community partners learn about one another. Your approach to these meetings is very important, as a dominant, self-centered approach will likely negatively impact future potential. Practice cultural humility and bring your listening skills. Academics can be viewed as aloof and even intimidating to community members. In CBPR, we need to break down these barriers and move toward equitable partnerships. The engagement process can be very time intensive and may take several years as the community learns to trust the researcher. Thus, for many early CBPR researchers, it may be easier to build on existing relationships established by successful CBPR researchers rather than starting from scratch. These investigators may be helpful in opening doors to the community and in vetting you as someone that can be trusted.

This needs assessment process is an important first step in developing a CBPR agenda, particularly if the researcher is unfamiliar with the community. Getting to know a community and those who are identified as leaders is step one in the engagement process. The process of meeting with individuals begins the foundational partnerships that are the basis of CBPR work. Community members have a chance to vet the researcher and vice versa. In communities where historical projects have left a distrust of research in general, this is particularly important. Why are you different from others? What will you provide for the community? How will this project benefit the citizens? This process can be challenging at first but is ultimately one of the most rewarding components of CBPR.

The data that a researcher obtains in this engagement process are instrumental for community mapping, that is, developing an in-depth understanding of the political organizational structure, the assets within the community, and the issues that concern community members. By identifying interpersonal connections, social networks, and the existing political landscape and infrastructure, one may also understand how things get done, what the opportunities for change are, and who can help sustain this change. Remember, CBPR is not only about the research itself but also about resulting action at the community level. In our Cambridge example, the researcher started with the data that had been collected over many years on schoolchildren's weight disparities. Along with a public health nutritionist and a doctoral student, she approached four longtime Cambridge colleagues who were considered "movers and shakers" in the Black community. These individuals had a commitment to the work and included a school principal, staff from the public health department, and a local nonprofit. They became "community investigators" on the project and, along with the researcher and public health nutritionist, identified themselves as the Healthy Eating and Living Project (H.E.L.P.) and began to investigate the underlying causes for the disparities. Through these relationships, the researcher was able to identify others who were not only concerned about the issue but were also likely to be able to make programmatic change. The success of the project relied heavily on this core of community investigators.

In the Somerville example, the engagement process took place at many levels. This included the mayoral level and other political and institutional leaders. It also included lay leaders in the community most affected by the suicides. And, finally, it included the youth who were friends of the deceased. Not all engagement proceeded at the same pace, and there were differing levels of trust. While the crisis demanded immediate teamwork, the relationships at the grassroots level—that is, the lay community leaders and the youth themselves—were the most difficult to establish. The researcher ended up in true partnership with the lay leaders but never developed strong partnerships with the youth, in part because this was ill advised, according to the lay community leaders. Instead, these leaders acted as liaisons, and the researcher did not push an alternative agenda. These lay leaders were pivotal advisors throughout the crisis.

In a similar fashion, most CBPR projects rely heavily on a community advisory board (CAB) or coalition that will participate in the research process and function as the liaison to the community. As you build your relationships, you should be thinking about who will serve on a community advisory group. The CAB will help to hone the research question and methodology and provide outreach to the population of interest as well as supply knowledge of local politics, pitfalls, and strategies. Choosing a group of community members to actively become part of your CAB is critical to the success of the project. Who are you working with? Are they committed to the project? Are they representative of the community of interest? Have you worked together previously and can you work together going forward? Do they want to be part of a CBPR project? What are the expectations for participation and how will information be communicated? In our Everett example, the community members who were already meeting were the natural CAB. In the Cambridge example, the researcher started with a community partner, and then, together, they identified and connected with other community members to form the advisory group. In our Somerville example, there was a task force that the mayor had convened, and this group served as the CAB for the investigation. Most CABs will meet regularly throughout the project. If grant dollars are available, they should be allocated to support this activity, including payment for community member time needed to participate.

Step 3: Refine the Research Question

Honing the research question starts with the topic of interest. In many cases, the community questions will be broad, reflecting timely concerns. "How do we stop drug abuse?" "Why is there youth violence?" "Why is autism increasing?" Community members are very helpful in identifying the topic of interest but may not have the skills to hone the research question. That is where the researcher's skills are most applicable. You should work with community partners to help focus the research questions. Your knowledge of the literature will help in this process, and by supplying the existing evidence, you can help the partnership consider what has already been discovered and think about new and emerging questions that have yet to be answered. Conduct a literature review and provide the important papers to the CAB. Part of your role is to educate the CAB about what is already known about the subject from a research perspective, just as the CAB will educate you about the subject from a community perspective. In our Everett example, the community asked if and how ICE was impacting immigrant health. The researchers identified prior literature on related subjects and provided this information to the group. This work also influenced the development of the conceptual framework. The final research questions were more nuanced than the original broad questions and included an exploration of how local police were perceived and whether ICE had an impact on health care access, on emotional well-being, or on chronic disease.

In the Somerville, Massachusetts example, in the midst of a health crisis, the community wanted to know how to stop the crisis. But first, it was important to understand how the crisis was proceeding. Was this a suicide cluster? Were the young people involved connected to one another? Was activity elevated over baseline? The researchers worked with the community to focus first on these questions and also to understand how other communities might have dealt with similar circumstances. The researcher plays an important role in translating the evidence into real-life situations. Similarly, in Cambridge, the questions were honed to a set of specific goals for the project: (A) understand the socio-demographic factors associated with obesity among Black school-aged children; (B) understand the social, cultural, and behavioral barriers and influences on diet and physical activity of Cambridge families; (C) identify a culturally relevant intervention to promote healthy weight in Black children and their families. This process of taking a community concern and reframing it into research questions and hypotheses is challenging. In Table 4.1, several examples are noted.

Table 4.1   Examples of Questions From Community and Researcher
Perspectives and Resulting Joint Hypotheses

Topic	Community Question	Investigator Question	Joint Hypothesis
• Youth violence	• How can we stop youth violence?	• What are the factors that are related to youth violence?	• Youth who have been incarcerated are more likely to be involved in violence within the first 6 months of release.
• Elderly falls	• Why are the elderly falling?	• Are there specific members of the elderly population who are at higher risks for falls?	• Elderly women living independently without spouses are more likely to fall than those in assisted living conditions.
• Adult obesity	• How can we stop obesity?	• Do obesity trends differ by gender, age, or race/ethnicity?	• Women are more likely to gain weight after their first pregnancy and continue to gain weight over time compared to women who have not had children, regardless of race/ethnicity.

Important First-Stage Considerations

- Learn about the community you are interested in through an informal needs assessment.
- Go into the community and meet people, begin conversations, get to know the culture.
- Work with a CAB to refine the questions for study.
- Serve as an educator and evidence translator.

❖ SECOND STAGE: DESIGN/HYPOTHESIS TESTING, ROLES
AND RESPONSIBILITIES, CONDUCT OF THE RESEARCH

Step 4: Design and Methods

Once there is consensus on a research question, the CAB and investigator should work together to frame the hypotheses to be tested and determine the best strategies for answering the research question. This will take place in a series of meetings of the CAB. While the investigator is likely to know more about the possible methods for investigation, the community partners possess the expertise to determine the feasibility of these methods. For example, even though an experimental approach may be the most valuable to answer the question, community members may have concerns regarding experimental methods due to other issues (time frames, access to participants, competing priorities). Community partners will need to reflect on how methods can or cannot be utilized and whether they are practical. In our Everett example, the initial work was exploratory in nature, and so methods that would allow for this type of exploration were chosen, including interviews, focus groups, and surveys. But while the investigators suggested that they hold several focus groups in only two languages so they could compare and contrast them, community members wanted to work with all the dominant language groups in their community in order to get a broad representation. The research team agreed to conduct six focus groups and changed its perspective to assess information across immigrant groups. So too, the researchers thought that documented and undocumented immigrants should be separated since they assumed these populations would have very different opinions on the topic. Community members felt this posed several problems. Undocumented immigrants were unlikely to come forward if they thought they would be singled out, and in many cases, families and social networks were made up of both documented and undocumented individuals. This information was then incorporated into the design. Research design required a negotiation in which the researcher introduced methods and community members considered the implications and practicality while also contributing real world evidence.

In our Somerville example, researchers identified methods for monitoring suicide and overdose activity while the crisis was occurring. This included examining death certificates and using 911 call data from the fire department. Community members were quick to point out that these sources had their own sets of problems. The death certificate data were often delayed if the body went to the medical examiner and the immediate cause of death was unknown. The 911 call data provided only initial impressions from the scene and did not provide follow-up of incidents. In turn, community members noted that youth were using websites to monitor cases themselves and introduced the researchers to these data sources, which provided information on connections of victims that was unknown to the CAB. As a result, researchers expanded their data collection to include website monitoring.

In the Cambridge example, parent/child interviews with local Black families were conducted. Conversations were held with various Black leadership groups (Men's Health League, Black Pastors Association) and parents and students at the high school and middle school. A survey of families at two schools was conducted. Introduction and access to these groups was provided by members of the CAB.

Step 5: Roles and Responsibilities

Once there is consensus on methods, roles and responsibilities for research conduct should be delineated. How will community partners participate in the research conduct? However, it is also important to remember that roles and responsibilities require financial resources, so prior to writing any grants, budgetary needs of both researcher and community member should be considered. In partnership, decide who will be involved in each step of the research process. This will be dependent to some extent on skills, expertise, and time. In the Everett project, community members were actively involved in tool development (focus group guides, surveys, and interview guides). They took the lead on focus group facilitation and participant recruitment. Researchers provided training sessions in focus group conduct and human subjects. Community members were less involved in analysis; they participated in initial identification of thematic content, and then researchers took over statistical and qualitative analysis. Results were presented to the CAB for interpretation and refinement.

In the Somerville example, community members led the task forces and researchers provided them with ongoing data for data-driven decisions. Then community members provided the context and the interpretation of the data. Community members were the main investigators when it came to outreach with youth, and researchers played more of a technical support role.

In the Cambridge example, the researcher and her team did the original quantitative analysis to understand some of the factors leading to disparities in BMI. The data were presented to the CAB in an iterative fashion, and CAB members assisted with interpretation. The CAB was also involved in designing all the tools for data collection, including interview guides and surveys, and members were involved in conducting the interviews. Throughout the entire project, the CAB members were intimately involved in the interpretation of the research findings.

Each of these examples demonstrates a slightly different approach to roles and responsibilities. However, it is important to recognize what partners bring to the table in the way of skills and expertise and build from there. Thinking through how the partnership will work throughout a project is an important part of the grant-writing and project development process. Transparent communication about expectations is also important, and using memoranda of agreement (MOA) or other strategies can be helpful to clearly articulate these expectations. Details of items to be included in an MOA are shown in Table 4.2.

Table 4.2   Components for a Memorandum of Agreement (MOA)

- Describe partners (who are the parties that are entering into this agreement?)
- Dates for MOA (beginning and end of project)
- Roles and responsibilities (who will actually do what; what each party agrees to do)
- Scope of work
- Timeline
- Deliverables (when and what is expected of each partner)
- Budget (how much, billing procedures)
- Publication rights and authorship
- Use of names of partners
- Data ownership (who owns data and how they can be used)

Step 6: Conduct Research

Conducting the research is largely dependent on preparation— that is, how well the roles and responsibilities were defined and how well procedures were outlined. In addition, adequate training is necessary to ensure accurate and complete data collection. There must also be a clear understanding of who is responsible for monitoring progress toward goals and dealing with unexpected events that can range from staff departures to ethical dilemmas to incomplete data. These responsibilities most often fall to the researchers but may be divided among community members as well. In the Everett example, community members were responsible for conducting the focus groups and taking notes. But the research team was responsible for ensuring that the dates for focus groups were set, that the community partners were trained in focus group conduct and ethics, and that notes were delivered in a timely fashion. While there were focus groups that lagged behind, frequent meetings of the CAB helped the project adhere to its timeline. A variety of tools to help in data collection and to decrease variability in data collection were developed, including templates for focus group notes, short surveys to collect first impressions after the focus groups, grids for analysis, and themes and scripts for interviews. In CBPR, academics and community partners are mutually dependent. The potential pitfalls are many. As is often the case, the researcher served as the overall principal investigator for the project and had ultimate responsibility for adhering to the institutional review board approval. In CBPR, regardless of who leads the project, there are many moving parts, which only increases the need for strong management. However, decisions are shared, and conflicts that arise during conduct will need to be collaboratively resolved.

In our Somerville example, all data were collected by the community. These data sources included the youth risk behavior survey that had been done annually and the 911 data, which were collected monthly by the fire department. The researchers analyzed and mapped the data. Community members also assisted with the examination of death certificate data. Today, in part as a result of this project, community members continue to collect these data for ongoing surveillance.

In our Cambridge example, secondary data on childhood obesity were collected by school physical education teachers, and the resulting dataset was used for analysis. Community members were involved in the development of all new data collection tools, and a community member joined a researcher for each of the parent/child interviews. The researcher, however, was responsible for the overall project and for moving the project forward.

There are many ways to engage the community in the conduct of CBPR. Their involvement in data collection can build their individual skills and the capacity of the community around data overall.

However, in a participatory process, management is required, and this is always harder when responsibilities are shared. The MOA plays an important role in setting the stage for CBPR, but it will be important to review progress regularly at CAB meetings, to deal with unexpected challenges, and to ensure the work gets done.

Second-Stage Considerations

- Work in partnership with community members to design the research and choose appropriate methods: balance rigor and practicality.
- Decide who is going to do what and make sure the resources are in place to get the work done.
- Monitor the conduct of the research, "make sure the trains are running on time," and develop strategies for addressing unexpected pitfalls.

❖ THIRD STAGE: ANALYSIS, INTERPRETATION, AND DISSEMINATION

Step 7: Analysis and Interpretation

Once roles have been clarified, think through the analysis and interpretation plan and discuss how both community members and researchers can be involved. In CBPR, it is not necessary that everyone is involved in everything to the same extent; however, it is important to recognize and address issues of data ownership. Remember, in CBPR, data ownership is something that should be negotiated up front, as data are not only the property of the researcher but also of the community partners. Negotiating decisions about how data will be used, when they can be shared with those external to the CAB, and who will house and "own" the data in the present and future will take some investment but will help solve potential future problems. Memoranda of agreement (see Table 4.2), referred to previously, can be helpful in documenting how these decisions should be made.

Roles in analysis often depend on expertise, time, and interest. For example, analyzing quantitative data using statistical methods is often best left to the researcher and the academic team, who have knowledge of statistical programs. However, there may be community members who want to learn more. In our Cambridge obesity example, the CAB decided on a preliminary analysis plan, that is, what variables they would explore and what statistical methods would be used. Then the researchers conducted analysis and brought frequencies back to the team prior to doing more extensive analysis to understand the questions that community members might observe. This assigning of meaning is one of the most important and valuable contributions of CBPR. The community partners will have an understanding of the context and meaning of these results. Their questions may be very different than those of the researchers. Their insight is extremely critical for later community action. Once additional decisions about analysis were made, the research team ran the analyses and once again brought it to the CAB. This iterative process helped to move the analysis forward in a manner that incorporated the multiple perspectives and enriched the end product. The CAB will be instrumental in interpreting results of any CBPR project as members bring their own understanding of the community issues to the process.

In our Somerville example, at the request of community partners, researchers took data from 911 calls and mapped them onto a map of Somerville using mapping software, and this revealed that certain areas of the community had higher levels of overdose and suicide activity than others. Community members could easily point out why these areas might have higher activity; for example, the area around a local college had a high level of alcohol 911 calls, while the area around the local housing project was known for drug activity. This information about the context of the community was particularly important in framing the meaning of the data and their interpretation. As a researcher involved in CBPR, recognizing what community members know about their community can be extremely helpful in this phase of the research.

Qualitative data may be somewhat more approachable than quantitative data for community partners. Listening to constituents is something that they do regularly. However, few are used to collecting and analyzing this type of data in a systematic manner, and it will be important to warn against jumping to conclusions based on one interview or focus group. The researcher can help facilitate the analysis of qualitative data by integrating community partners into the process. Again, this can be an iterative process, with initial work being done by the researcher and then presented to the CAB for refinement, reanalysis, and presentation again until all are satisfied with the codebook. This was the process undertaken with the focus groups in the Everett example. After completion of the focus groups, the CAB identified initial themes. Then the data were entered into a software package and further categorized, then presented to the CAB and modified and reanalyzed again. The process took about 3 months but benefited from the multiple perspectives of both researchers and CAB members. In short, while analysis may seem a cumbersome process to share between researcher and community, it can be done through creative strategies that ultimately enrich the process and improve the relevancy of the work.

Step 8: Dissemination

Lastly, the dissemination of results as a final step in the CBPR process often takes multiple forms. As a researcher, you are likely to be interested in peer-reviewed journals, while community partners are much more likely to want immediate dissemination so that they can utilize the results in action. This can present many conflicts for researcher and community alike. For example, in Everett, the community wanted a forum at which results could be presented and recommendations discussed. The researchers wanted to produce a paper for publication and were concerned about how release of data would impact their ability to publish. They agreed on a compromise that resulted in several strategies. First, a large community forum with a PowerPoint presentation of the high-level results was presented in a digestible form at the end of the project. Community members took the lead on orchestrating the forum, including the invitation list, the food, and the space. The researchers took the lead on the initial draft of the presentation, and then the PowerPoint was circulated among all partners for critique and edits. The forum also had an interactive component in which community members had a chance to develop recommendations for action based on the presentation. The list of recommendations was finalized and presented to institutional leaders (mayor, police chief, and schools). Advocacy agencies took the recommendations and incorporated them into their activities. Simultaneously, the researcher developed an outline for a peer-reviewed paper and asked all those on the CAB if they wanted to be authors. Authorship brought responsibilities, including some editing and writing. Not everyone wanted to participate, but over the course of the next year, all the authors (there were 10 in total) had a chance to review drafts, comment, and provide feedback. Two papers from the project were accepted for publication. The community, meanwhile, acted on some of the recommendations. They began meeting with local police to address traffic stops, which changed the dynamics between the immigrant community and the police overall. Almost a year later, the police were no longer "arresting" people who did not have driver's licenses. Instead, they would issue citations. This meant that undocumented immigrants were able to avoid fingerprinting and reporting to ICE. The police/immigrant relations improved as regular meetings with police were held. One immigrant advocacy leader noted that the number of complaints about police from the immigrant community had fallen dramatically.

Dissemination in the Cambridge example was handled somewhat differently but with similar attributes. A formal report was made to the chief public health officer for the city and to the CAB. A final written report was drafted and vetted by community partners.[4] In turn, this was presented to other Cambridge leaders to get their perspectives on potential action steps. The CAB was able to obtain some additional funding to maintain its work as it applied for additional funds to pilot test an intervention.

Overall, the dissemination process should be considered in two simultaneous manners: that is, what and how to disseminate results for the benefit of the community members while also publishing results in peer-reviewed journals for generalizability. Both academic and community partners are driven by real incentives, and these end products highlight the differences between them. While these two agendas can conflict, there are ways in which both parties can be satisfied and gain from the process. The two dissemination strategies may also have different timelines; the community may want immediate results that can be utilized in practical applications at either the policy or programmatic level. The time for article production may be much longer and somewhat irrelevant to the community but important to the researcher. Straddling these potentially conflicting goals is difficult, but as long as communication is open and transparent, the dissemination process can flow smoothly and obstacles can be addressed. There is no question that group dissemination is cumbersome, but the differing perspectives enrich the final products and make them not only more relevant to the community but also more likely to have sustainable outcomes and a "life" after the CBPR project is completed.

Identifying action steps is really in the hands of the community partners. While it is part of the dissemination process, the researcher may or may not be involved. However, the researcher can play an important role in sustaining the CBPR collaboration. In our three examples, action steps resulting from the CBPR projects included the following:

1. Everett: regular meetings held with immigrants and police to enhance communication; health care providers improved awareness how ICE affects their immigrant patients.

2. Somerville: regular monitoring of 911 activity; development of a citywide trauma response network.

3. Cambridge: recommendations developed for future interventions, including: encourage youth to drink water, expand programming for Black girls to be physically active, limit TV consumption, and avoid using food to comfort children when they are upset.

Third-Stage Considerations

- Determine how partners will be involved in both analysis and interpretation.
- Use an iterative process to assign meaning and generate consensus on that meaning.
- Utilize multiple dissemination strategies important to both community members and academics.
- Identify action steps.

❖ CONCLUSION

In summary, there are clear steps in the CBPR process that should be considered (see Table 4.3). Engagement of the community, defining the questions, conducting the research, and disseminating findings all take time and should be addressed in a participatory manner. The CAB provides an excellent organizing strategy for working with community partners, but the research team of community members and academics must map out communication and roles and responsibilities and conduct the study in an environment of mutual respect.

Table 4.3   Summary of CBPR Steps

Stage 1
Community Engagement[5-7]

- Identify the community of interest.
- Conduct a needs assessment to understand the issues for potential research.
- Meet the stakeholders.
- Develop relationships.
- Assemble a CAB.
- Choose an area for research.
- Conduct a literature review.
- Hone the research questions and hypotheses.

Stage 2
Research Design, Roles, and Responsibilities

- Discuss methods.
- Assess feasibility.
- Define roles for community and for researcher.
- Provide education and skill development.
- Conduct study.

Stage 3
Analysis, Interpretation, and Dissemination

- Assess skills.
- Develop iterative processes.
- Work with CAB for interpretation and context.
- Determine dissemination modes.
- Develop processes that allow all to participate.
- Identify action steps based on evidence.

❖ QUESTIONS AND ACTIVITIES

The purpose of this assignment is to help students put ideas about CBPR into practice. If you can actually assign your students to work with local community partners, you can provide them with real-world experience. If that is not an option, have them work in groups to develop a CBPR research proposal that addresses one of the community health problems described below (i.e., childhood obesity, youth suicide, disparities in mortality among women living with HIV, or disparities in cardiovascular disease among Black men).

Guidance

1. Describe your CBPR approach.

2. Who are your community partners and how will you engage them?

3. What is your research design?
   - Sample
   - Recruitment
   - Methods
   - Analysis (optional)

4. How will you disseminate findings? What will you do with the findings?

5. Identify potential challenges or limitations.

Scenario 1—Youth Suicide

Community Context

Setting: a community that is suburban with a population of about 80,000. The suburb is fairly wealthy, with average home costs hovering around $500,000. It has a reasonable tax base and is home to an outstanding university, where you work. The population is by and large White, and there is not much diversity economically, but the population is changing as educated South Asians move into the community.

Description of a health problem: In 2010, one teenager who was attending the local high school committed suicide via a pill overdose. Within several months, her best friend also left a note, and she too committed suicide, but she jumped from a building in the downtown area. Parents of high school children are in an uproar, demanding that the school do something to prevent another suicide. Teens are holding vigils for their lost friends.

Partners That Came to You With the Problem

Members of the school committee have convened a task force of parents, teachers, and members of the local churches.

Health Question

What is happening in their community that could be leading to such a situation? They also want to understand if these two suicides represent a "cluster" or "contagious" situation. They feel they need this information to inform their next steps.

Scenario 2—Cardiovascular Disease in Men

Community Context

This is a city in the Midwest of about 1 million. There has been a real economic downturn here, and the unemployment rate is upward of 10%. There is a large Black population in one area of the city, which is also an area with high rates of poverty and even higher rates of unemployment.

Health Problem

The rates of stroke and heart attacks in the Black male population are alarming and far outstrip those for Whites in the city. There are two hospitals, one catering to the small economically well-off population and one that is the "poverty" hospital.

Partners That Came to You With the Problem

Providers at the poverty hospital have seen ever-increasing rates of young men coming in with strokes. They want to do something to change the situation, but many men do not seek health care in part because they are uninsured and unemployed.

Health Question

How can the health care system identify and reach out to men of color who are at risk for cardiovascular disease?

Scenario 3—Childhood Obesity

Community Context

This is a middle-income city on the West Coast with a population of approximately 100,000 persons. Approximately 30% of the population is under the age of 18, the majority of whom attend public schools across the city. The city is racially and ethnically diverse. There is a large immigrant community from Mexico and other Central American countries. There is also a growing Southeast Asian population.

Health Problem

In 2004, all of the city's schools began measuring students' BMI and reporting back to parents the results of the assessment. Educational materials have been sent home with the reports, and school nurses are available to follow up with parents who are interested in learning more about what they can do to improve their children's health. Since 2004, BMI scores have steadily increased among every racial and ethnic group in the city. BMI scores are particularly high in several elementary schools.

Partners That Came to You With the Problem

The PE teacher in one school with particularly high BMI scores among students came to you with the data the school has been collecting over the last few years. The PE teacher has been in touch with the school's family council, PTA, teachers, and administrators.

Potential Health Questions

Why are BMI scores increasing at a higher rate among students in some schools? What underlies the increase in BMI scores?

Questions

1. What are some of the factors to consider in engaging community partners in analysis of data?

2. How does the process of dissemination differ in a CBPR project from a non-CBPR process?

3. In what ways would community partners use data from a CBPR project to take action?

❖ NOTES

1.   Hacker K, Chu J, Leung C, Marra R, Pirie A, Brahimi M, English M, Beckmann J, Acevedo-Garcia D, Marlin RP. The impact of Immigration and Customs Enforcement on immigrant health: perceptions of immigrants in Everett, Massachusetts, USA. *Social Science & Medicine*. 2011 Aug;73(4):586–94.

2.   Hacker K, Collins J, Gross-Young L, Almeida S, Burke N. Coping with youth suicide and overdose: one community's efforts to investigate, intervene, and prevent suicide contagion. *Crisis.* 2008;29(2):86–95.

3.   U.S. Census Bureau. *2006–2008 American Community Survey 3-Year Estimates.* 2008 [cited 2010 October 3]; Available from http://factfinder2.census.gov.

4.   Chomitz V, Arsenault L, Banks C, et al. *H.E.L.P. Culminating Report.* Cambridge, MA: Institute for Community Health; 2011.

5.   Clinical and Translational Science Awards Consortium. Community Engagement Key Function Committee Task Force on the Principles of Community Engagement. *Principles of Community Engagement.* 2nd ed. Rockville, MD: NIH; 2011.

6.   Israel BA, Parker EA, Rowe Z, et al. Community-based participatory research: lessons learned from the Centers for Children's Environmental Health and Disease Prevention Research. *Environmental Health Perspectives.* 2005 Oct; 113(10):1463–71.

7.   Minkler M, Wallerstein N., eds. *Community-Based Participatory Research for Health.* San Francisco, CA: Jossey-Bass; 2003.

5

Translating Research Into Practice

View From Community

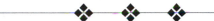

"Sustainability is building capacity and helping the community use their own data to help them continue work after the intervention has finished." (Community partner-conference participant)[1]

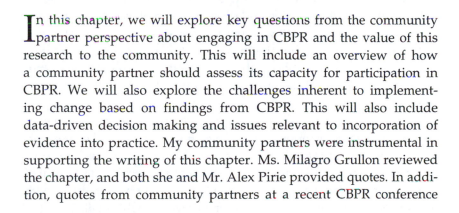

In this chapter, we will explore key questions from the community partner perspective about engaging in CBPR and the value of this research to the community. This will include an overview of how a community partner should assess its capacity for participation in CBPR. We will also explore the challenges inherent to implementing change based on findings from CBPR. This will also include data-driven decision making and issues relevant to incorporation of evidence into practice. My community partners were instrumental in supporting the writing of this chapter. Ms. Milagro Grullon reviewed the chapter, and both she and Mr. Alex Pirie provided quotes. In addition, quotes from community partners at a recent CBPR conference on building community capacity were also used.[1] The coalitions that I worked with in the given examples approved the use of their stories.

The following fictional example helps to illustrate a typical community response to a researcher request.

> I am the executive director of a small organization dedicated to serving the Latino community in Community Y. We are currently fairly small, with only two employees. All of us are immigrants and speak fluent Spanish. The mission of our organization is to provide help with access to health care, city services, and other programs for the Latino immigrant community. A researcher from the local university has contacted us and wants to get our help recruiting Latinos for a study on mental health issues. In the past, we had a bad experience with a researcher. He asked for our help recruiting our constituents for a study on high blood pressure. We spent more than a month helping with the recruitment, and while we did get paid for our efforts, our small staff could not do this work and keep up with the work of the organization. Things were very tense. Then, when he completed the research, we never heard back from him about the results until we read them in the newspaper. "Latino males who are overweight are at high risk for hypertension." We never had a chance to participate in the paper or get the results so we could work with the community to improve the situation. It was a surprise to us and to the people who had agreed to participate. Overall, it felt like we got used, and we are not sure we want to do this again.

In the world of community research, this is not an uncommon situation. What went wrong? There was money shared, and engagement seems to have taken place, but things really seem to have fallen down in the analysis/interpretation and dissemination phase of the research. In this case, it is hard to tell whether the researcher was interested in a full CBPR relationship, but the impact of this research has ultimately increased the divide between the community and researchers, and, most importantly, while it may have contributed to the literature, it has provided little benefit to the local community.

Many community partners may have negative impressions of research influenced by prior historical events such as the Tuskegee experiment, especially in communities of color. They may have had negative experiences with past research projects themselves and feel distrustful of new academic relationships. Additionally, they may be unfamiliar with how research works or what their role in this work might entail.

"Communities have no motivation because these research projects go on yet there is no investment in the community after. Many community members are not interested in being in a registry for research." (Community partner-conference participant)[1]

"There is this mistrust of what the aims are for research and what this information will be used for." (Community partner-conference participant)[1]

Recognizing that these perspectives may linger long past any one individual research project is an important part of the engagement process. A researcher needs to be aware of the history of research in the community. Community partners need to be empowered to ask the hard questions of researchers so as not to repeat the same mistakes. They need to understand the benefits and pitfalls of engaging in research. Gaining this insight is part of the engagement process and is necessary for the development of a strong CBPR partnership. As a community begins to understand research and its potential power, community members may initiate CBPR projects themselves, recognizing that they need data to catalyze social change in policy and practice.

In our previous Everett example, Everett, one member of an immigrant advocacy group acknowledged the potential benefit of engaging in research. As a member of a community advocacy group dedicated to working with Latinos in Everett, he was very concerned about how recent immigration enforcement activity was affecting the Latino community. Immigrant activists had many stories of how immigrants were being stopped and asked for their driver's licenses, and then, if they did not have a license, they were arrested. Many immigrants were in fear of their safety, suspecting that this action would result in deportation. The immigrant advocacy community wanted to get more information on this situation to convince the police to stop arresting people for not having a valid driver's license. They had made a connection with a local researcher that they already knew and trusted when a grant opportunity arose. They asked her to help them get the data needed to actively change the situation. In this example, the Everett community partners recognized that data collected through "research" might help them advocate for action. This academic/community partnership was built on an existing trusting relationship.[2] While not all CBPR partnerships will be initiated by the community and all questions will not be solely originated in the community, using a CBPR approach resets the researcher's agenda such that the topic of study resonates with community priorities and is seen as beneficial to the community. Community members should expect that their priorities will be considered and that their perspectives will be valued in the research agenda and subsequent process.

❖ ASSESSING COMMUNITY RESEARCH READINESS

"How do you justify this money being spent on research? Communities have real issues that money could help solve and yet this money is being given to research—how do you prove the benefit and then share the money so that it benefits the community (immediately)?" (Community member-conference participant)[1]

As noted previously (Chapter 2), it is important to assess the impact that engaging in research will have on the community. The areas outlined below are important for community members to address prior to engaging in a CBPR project.

❖ ASSESSING THE PARTNERSHIP

The first area that community partners will need to assess is the nature of the CBPR partnership itself, the values, goals, and priorities.[3] What type of partnership is planned? How much power will the community members have in decision making? Is the researcher intimidating? Is he or she skilled in participatory techniques? Does she or he speak in layman's terms and understand the community perspective? Is there a history of trust and respect?[4] Is the researcher's agenda shared by the community?

"Today, decisions are made by prioritizing and based upon the needs in the community. From a program perspective we need research to help implement the correct programs in our community. Prioritizing according to need can yield rich data to support programs and interventions. Again, what makes a project appealing is the need and if the community has identified what is being presented as a priority for them." Milagro Grullon, Lawrence, MA

In order to learn more about the researchers, their goals, background, and expectations of a partnership, a face-to-face meeting should be held, and community members should have a chance to ask these questions and determine if the CBPR project is right for them. Questions outlined in Table 5.1 are a good place to start. In addition, the city of Lawrence, Massachusetts, developed a "tools for research partnerships" document that can help community partners build their formal agreements with researchers.[5] As one partner noted related to the choice of an academic partner:

"Is this a person you can spend the next year or four years working with closely? Is she or he someone you can comfortably disagree with? Are they sympathetic to the complexities and nuances of communities and willing to step outside of their traditional bubbled and siloed turf to connect with the community?" Alex Pirie, Somerville, MA

Table 5.1   Questions for Community Partners

Questions for community partners to ask researcher prior to engaging in CBPR

1. What kind of partnership does the researcher have in mind? Is it really to be participatory?
2. How will decisions get made?
3. What are the research aims?
4. Who is the target population of interest?
5. How will the research be funded?
6. What will be our organization's and/or my role in the project?
7. Will the time be compensated?
8. Who will own the data? What will happen to the data in the future after the project is completed?
9. What benefits will the project leave behind in the community (skills, programming, policy, infrastructure, capacity building)?
10. What is the dissemination plan for this research?
11. Does the researcher have the skills and experience to collaborate?
12. Does he or she understand the complexity of the CBPR approach?
13. Does the researcher possess cultural humility?

Questions for community partners to ask themselves prior to engaging in CBPR

1. Does this study address an important problem relevant to my community and my constituents?
2. How does the research aim fit with the mission of my organization?
3. Do we have the capacity to participate? Space? Staff? Time?
4. What are our conflicting priorities?
5. What will be the impact of doing research on my organization's ability to get its core work accomplished?
6. Will the results lead to action that will help my community?

❖ TIME, RESOURCES, AND CAPACITY

As part of the development of a partnership pre–CBPR, community members should ask specific questions in three critical areas to assess their own readiness for research: time, money, and capacity. That is, do they have the time to participate without sacrificing their other responsibilities, are they going to get appropriate financial resources from the researcher to support their work, and do they have the organizational capacity to participate in the research project? Each of these issues can create problems if resources are inadequate for the project. For example, if the organization and the staff do not have time available to participate in the CAB meetings or to actually conduct their roles in the research, they will be unable to fulfill their responsibilities and the research will fail. As one community member said:

> "The single largest obstacle to collaborations between academic and community partners is time. The relative time frames of academic and community partners can create huge problems and it is essential that whichever of the two sides of the partnership is more experienced do everything it can to educate the other on the discontinuity that exists." Alex Pirie, Somerville, MA

In many organizations, particularly small ones, it is not feasible to just hire additional people to take on the new work of a research project. So who will do the work? What are the implications for the organization? In addition, there is time required to participate in CBPR partnership meetings and time required for the development of proposals and dissemination products. Finally, sometimes, it can take several years before a research grant is funded. Any community partner must consider where it will be in the future and whether it is able to plan that far in advance.

Where the money is concerned, budgets should reflect an equitable process between community and academic partners. Community partners have not always been included in these decisions.

> "When I first started working with academic institutions (12 years ago) I had no involvement with budgets. I was given an amount for participating as a [representative of the] community without being asked how many staff would be involved or the hours we

would spend on the project. We realized shortly after the grant started that the demands on the staff and community were greater than the funds could sustain." Milagro Grullon, Lawrence, MA

As one prepares a grant proposal, both community and academic participants should assess whether there is adequate support for a CBPR project. Financial support is needed for items ranging from community coinvestigators, liaisons, space, meetings, and advisors to travel and dissemination. It should reflect the division of labor between academics and the community.

"Depending on the involvement and time spent in the research, resources should be divided accordingly. The community is asked to participate and do a lot of work (meetings, gather data, interviews, invite community members, go on the radio, etc. etc.). Without the community, some of the research could not take place. Researchers need the community, and the community needs to get paid justly." Milagro Grullon, Lawrence, MA

Table 5.2 shows an example of a CBPR budget for a project that included focus groups and surveys. The dollars for various items (stipends, food, etc.) can either sit with the academic or the community partner, depending in large part on their ability to distribute the money. In some cases, community organizations may see a CBPR project as a way of accessing dollars for needed infrastructure and programming. However, the research dollars are not flexible and cannot be spent on nonresearch-related items. Regardless of how the ultimate budget looks, it should be negotiated up front, and any further reductions that might be required if the grant is funded should also be discussed with the partnership prior to starting the project.

Ms. Grullon recalled:

"The second time around, when an institution came to me for help or to develop a (pseudo) partnership, I started making clear demands. I needed to see the budget and be included just as any researcher would be listed on the budget. I worked on a budget for the organization and the community members that would be involved." Milagro Grullon, Lawrence, MA

Table 5.2   Proposed CBPR Project Budget

	FTE	Salary	Fringe	Request
Academic Institution				
Principal investigator	0.1	—	—	
Research associate	0.5	—	—	
Data analyst	0.2	—	—	
Stipends for community advisory group	5 per	$50/per		$2,500
Focus group stipends for participants	16 per	$25/per		$400
Incentives for surveys	100 per	$5		$500
Translation costs	1000 words	$.15/word		$150
Transcription	2	$250/ea		$500
Community Contract				
Community co-investigator	0.2	—	—	
Research assistants	0.5	—	—	
Stipends for focus group facilitators	$50 per	2 focus groups with 8 persons each		$800
Space				$250
Office supplies				$250
Food for two focus groups		$100/per		$200

Source: Reproduced by permission from Institute for Community Health, Inc. Cambridge, MA 2011 www.icommunityhealth.org

While differences in salary ranges can become a source of conflict, a bigger issue for many community partners is the high rates of indirect costs that most academic institutions claim. This can be a source of great tension in CBPR. "Indirect" rates are related to costs that include physical plant, research administration, and so forth, and they are negotiated with the funding institution. As one community member said:

"When people congratulate us and say, 'wow, you got a million bucks to study X, Y, or Z!,' I say, well, no, we got about 45% of that, the rest goes to mow lawns and trim ivy at the University of Wherever." Alex Pirie, Somerville, MA

In general, these dollars do not flow directly to the principal investigator but, rather, are used by the institution to support operations. While some community agencies have successfully negotiated an indirect rate with funders, this is not always the case. Thus, how they support their operational needs (rent, secretarial support, utilities, and payroll) comes into question. A community organization needs to discuss strategies for covering these costs with the researcher either as an indirect rate, if allowed, or by putting these items into direct costs. Without these transparent negotiations, the budget can become a major source of conflict.

The capacity of the community partner may include things like current staffing, financial health (cash flow, total budget, grant management skills), and physical space. For example, can the organization accommodate the research given its personnel issues (turnover rates, skill sets, etc.)? Are there procedures in place to deal with contracts? Is there enough cash flow to conduct the work and then invoice for work done? How will the research impact the day-to-day operations of the organization? Any community partner or member of a community organization should consider these issues prior to agreeing to participate in a CBPR project.

It is also important to remember that research is relatively inflexible compared to program implementation. This "rigidness" is needed to answer the research questions effectively. If the intervention keeps changing or the staff leaves and new staff must be retrained, it poses a problem for the research. Data need to be collected on every participant in a consistent manner. Records about why participants did not participate as well as how many did or did not participate must be maintained. If a survey is done but no one knows what the total number of potential participants in the target group was, it will be impossible to calculate the response rate. While these may be seemingly simple steps, in practice they can be a major challenge. In the Everett project, surveys of community doctors were done, but the process of figuring out exactly how many community doctors were serving Everett populations turned out to be much more complicated than expected. Community partners wanted to send the survey out to as many providers as possible to generate a high number of responses, but researchers first needed to figure out how many providers were serving the Everett community. In other words, they needed to know the denominator so that they could understand whether the final sample was representative of the total group of providers. A similar situation happened when community partners wanted to survey immigrants. They held several forums and passed out surveys but were unable to keep track of who refused to fill out the survey or even how many potential participants were at the forum. Researchers found themselves counting attendees and trying to keep track of who got surveys, who filled them out, and who threw them in the waste-basket. In the end, they were unable to determine what percentage of attendees actually did fill out the surveys.

Sampling concepts may be foreign to community groups, who may have little experience with obtaining responses in a systematic way. The tension between action and rigor may create conflict with the organization's culture and capacity. After all, communities do not exist in a laboratory bubble. Unexpected events transpire that may have a deep impact on a research project, ranging from turnover in local leadership to new and emerging social issues. Service demand may interfere with scientific methodology. While not all research will require the same level of rigor, adherence to a protocol really matters. For community partners, this may present a very different approach to conducting business. The research will need to get done on schedule to achieve the aims set out in the proposal. CBPR is often a balancing act between the researcher's need for control to achieve scientifically valid results and the community's desire for action. Successful CBPR partnerships are able to navigate these challenges via mindful communication and planning.

❖ DATA COLLECTION, OWNERSHIP, AND PROTECTION

"Data is not a four-letter word. Advancing the field and advancing the science [will only happen] because we have done good research and then it will help." (Community partner-conference participant)[1]

Data and their collection, security, use, and ownership is an area that requires some forethought in CBPR. Given that CBPR represents a partnership for both community and academics, the data are the property of both. How they are handled, analyzed, and disseminated is therefore important for both. As noted in previous chapters, some of these issues can be sorted out and recorded in a memorandum of agreement. In our Somerville CBPR youth suicide example, the researchers were helpful in translating real-time data into usable information for community partners. They provided the analytic capacity to examine the youth risk behavior data and identified additional data sources that were useful in monitoring suicide and overdose activity. These included death certificate data, 911 call data from the fire department, and hospital data on use of the emergency room related to suicide intention and overdose. They were able to provide these enhanced data to the community for real-time decision making. In addition, they were able to map data from the 911 call information onto maps of the community. This helped provide a contextual framework that allowed community members to focus their attention on specific areas. The data were generally "deidentified," meaning that information that would identify a person was removed before reporting to the CAB. No one would be able to identify the individuals, thus maintaining their privacy. The concept of data privacy is an important one in CBPR. Working with community members who may know each other could put privacy at risk. In CBPR, it is particularly important to work through these privacy issues prior to sharing data. In Somerville, the CAB agreed to a level of privacy that would not allow reporting when numbers were small (< 5).[6]

The Somerville project is an example of using data for decision making in real time. While community members bring a wealth of tacit knowledge to the table, they are not always equipped to evaluate their efforts. Thus, the ability to use and analyze data in a more rigorous fashion may help to promote improvement. In CBPR, data can serve both as means to a research project end and as quality-improvement information for community partners. As noted, the translation of evidence to everyday practical solutions is a critical component of the CBPR process. The CBPR researcher is, in effect, a purveyor of data, design, and methods that will facilitate this translation. Key to this translation are the skills to communicate and the desire to utilize. The CBPR research process resembles the Plan Do Study Act cycle in quality improvement.

To a community partner, the collection and management of these data thus have implications for the present project but also, potentially, for future programmatic and policy decisions. Community partners should be very thoughtful about how the data will be housed and about how decisions about present and future analysis will be handled. The misuse of data can seriously undermine any future research efforts and potentially fracture a CBPR partnership. Setting out strict standards about data use at the beginning of the project can be beneficial. Table 5.3 is an example of an explicit policy regarding data confidentiality. This will be discussed at length in the next chapter.

Table 5.3   Data Ownership and Confidentiality[7]

There should be an explicit agreement between researchers and community and university partners with respect to ownership of the research data. The nature of the agreement will be determined on a project-by-project basis, as the community needs/requirements may differ (i.e., a school, a department of health, and a coalition may require different agreements). This agreement should be made prior to the onset of the project and revisited during the project with the project-specific working group.

Research projects will adhere to the human subjects review process standards and procedures set forth by the appropriate institutional review board. In addition, research partners will adhere to standards of school departments and community-based organizations when appropriate.

All investigators and research associates need to be certified for human subjects work.

All persons who work with data (including visiting scholars and graduate students) will be required to sign a pledge of confidentiality for data use.

In general, we will not publicly report data with a cell size less than 5 subjects. Suppression of cell sizes < 5 in reporting will be considered the general rule to protect the confidentiality of subjects. However, any agreement requiring larger numbers for suppression will supersede this rule.

Source: Institute for Community Health, Cambridge, MA 2012.

❖   DISSEMINATION OF FINDINGS

"The time delay between the conclusion of a research project and the publication of papers is always a problem. This is a period of time when, because of the constraints of journal publication, there is a virtual embargo on the results except in the most general way, and it drives the community side nuts. 'Hey, we know this, we want to do something with/about it!'" Alex Pirie, Somerville, MA

Identifying the results of CBPR research is the first step in translating evidence into actionable efforts. As is part of the CBPR process, the community is generally interested in using the results to make change. Change can be actualized in many forms: new programs to address needs, changes in existing programs, policy change at the local and state levels, and advocacy efforts. Findings make their way into these venues in multiple fashions. Program directors that have access to the information can incorporate it into their day-to-day work. Advocates can promote the results with their city councilors, aldermen, and legislatures to move an agenda forward; constituents can use the evidence to improve their own situations. This is one of the most important value-added benefits of participating in CBPR efforts.

"Don't save dissemination [or evidence] translation until the end. Systemic changes are key. Wait for results of qualitative + quantitative research to see what worked and let the community know. Policy + systemic changes has built sustainability. Make it a priority to have dialogue with community [and] key stakeholders." (Community member-conference participant)[1]

In all research, the findings are not always what one might expect. Sometimes, results do not reveal the answers that one is seeking, or they reveal unexpected information that may be particularly controversial. How will the partnership deal with conflictual and potentially controversial results? Will community members want to censure the results? Will they want to reframe the discussion? Community partners need to be prepared for these possibilities and discuss how they will deal with results in advance of their delivery. In CBPR, the community partners are part of the analysis and interpretation phase of the research, and this will help in the management of the dissemination process because of their involvement in interpretation. However, from a community perspective, if you go into a project to prove something or to demonstrate how well your program works, you may be disappointed. Community partners need to be realistic about what the research can provide and discuss various possibilities for how they will deal with positive, negative, or neutral results with their academic partners well in advance of fielding the research.

The definition of *dissemination* may be very different for academics and community partners. Community partners want to get the information into the hands of policy makers or service providers in the form of reports, press coverage, or community meetings. In our Everett example, the community partners requested that data be presented to the community in a public forum at the end of the project so that community members could make recommendations for action. They were adamant that this needed to happen quickly so as not to lose the momentum of the project. In addition, given the focus of the work, the timing regarding the larger context of immigration enforcement was opportune. The researchers would have to wait to work on publications for peer-reviewed journals until after this was done. Together, they decided to present the data in a digestible format to an audience convened by the community partners, who included local government as well as immigrants themselves. They also requested that community members have an opportunity to consider recommendations for action based on the study. This engagement was built into the forum agenda. Participants broke up into different language groups and worked together to answer key questions and provide recommendations. The final product was a set of policy and practice recommendations that was provided to leaders in the community. Many were then utilized to change police-immigrant relationships and address health care access issues.[2] Afterward, the researcher and community partners developed several papers for peer-reviewed journals. The emphasis for dissemination was different for community and academics. Several other dissemination options were also used that particularly spoke to advocacy, including a press release to local papers, a letter to the *Boston Globe,* and several submissions to pertinent blogs. The dissemination plan for the project has since taken multiple forms.

- Community forum with presentation
- Meetings with advocacy groups
- Meetings with police
- Presentations to local community advisory group
- Abstracts at national meetings
- Peer-reviewed publication(s)
- Press release(s)
- Letters to newspapers
- Blog submissions

❖ TRANSLATION OF EVIDENCE INTO PRACTICE

"We always have to examine whether or not we are doing what we hope to be doing. But this is difficult because we get invested in what we are doing and taking a critical examination is not always easy." (Community member-conference participant)[1]

Dissemination of study results jump-starts the process of translation/adoption of evidence into practice. As people hear about the ideas, they are likely to consider how to implement them. In addition, if the findings are strong, they may influence how programs are run and, more importantly, whether programs continue to exist. Some of the decisions about translation and sustainability may depend on the project topic. For example, if community members wanted to test an intervention, there may already be tacit agreement to adopt the findings, when available, or to change or adapt the program to improve it. The CBPR process is also making all kinds of new evidence available, including literature reviews, information on evidence-based practices, and existing data for use in this CBPR process. There are often unexpected outcomes of CBPR that may not have been the primary focus but are results of multidisciplinary approaches that start with academic/community partnerships. Certainly, if adoption is contingent on money, translation and sustainability might be harder to achieve. But the results of one study provide the foundation for the next. In Everett, the community took the results and translated them directly into actionable steps. They launched police/immigrant meetings. But they also used the data to obtain additional grants on racism and food insecurity and adolescent risk behaviors. The data continue to have a life after the project. In Somerville, the community continued its vigilance by monitoring 911 activity after the suicide/overdose crisis. They hired a mental health coordinator who is still in place. In Cambridge, the work is ongoing, and the partners have written several other grants. While the project provides new data for communities, it also shapes the researchers and their agendas. They benefit greatly from the colearning of the partnership.

Overall, community partners should expect any CBPR researcher to be aware of the impact of a CBPR project on a community at all different phases. This includes the impact on community partner capacity, mission, and time. Researchers should recognize from the beginning that shared goals for a project need to be discussed and mutually decided. Dissemination strategies take many forms, and communities perceive action—local action—as an end product. A CBPR researcher should understand what the incentives for community participation are and simultaneously acknowledge her or his own. Thus, as a final portion of this chapter, we offer a list of questions that a researcher should consider prior to CBPR engagement.

Researcher Questions to Answer Before Getting Involved in CBPR

- Is my question emanating from community priorities?
- Will the results or findings of this study benefit the community?
- What am I really asking from the community partners? What level of responsibility will the community bear?
- How do I ensure that my partners understand the research and its limitations, the benefits and risks?
- Can I frame multiple dissemination products to serve both my goals and those of my community partners?
- Am I in it for the long haul? What is my commitment to the community?

A researcher who puts him- or herself in the community's shoes and understands the community's perspective will go a long way toward supporting the CBPR process and improving the level of trust in community/academic relationships.

"The strategy is to form it [the research] around a very clear, specific issue that everyone feels invested in. Then you can start building the trust and relationship." (Community member-conference participant)[1]

❖ CONCLUSION

Community partners who wish to engage in CBPR should be aware of the benefits as well as the challenges of this approach. They should be thoughtful about their own research readiness and aware of the realities—the responsibilities and the potential outcomes—of engaging in a research project. They should seek a balanced partnership in which their voice is heard and their viewpoints considered. Most importantly, they should consider how the outcomes of CBPR will help their community, however that is defined. Knowledge is powerful. CBPR is an approach to gaining knowledge that can empower communities. Thus, a well-designed CBPR study is more likely to encourage strong, trusting relationships that cross academic/community boundaries and improve the translation of both evidence-based practice and practice-based evidence into practical solutions for real-life problems.

❖ QUESTIONS AND ACTIVITIES

Activities

Have students break up into small groups to discuss the following:

A community group had garnered a grant to develop and implement a program for African American men to improve cardiovascular risk factors. The program was well liked by participants and by local politicians. But they had no idea if the program made a difference in participants' health. Initial data were promising with regard to satisfaction and engagement of the participants, but there was no evidence that the outcomes (BP, cholesterol) were changing. There was a great deal of investment in the program, and a publication that did not say "the program was working" would put the program at risk financially. They engaged a local CBPR researcher to work with them and try to evaluate the impact of the project.

What are the potential pitfalls in taking on this project?

Describe the community perspective and their incentives underlying this work.

How would you disseminate results?

What types of products might bring added value to the community?

Have students interview other CBPR researchers to ask them about their projects and how they approached the steps or a particular step outlined in this chapter.

If possible, have students sit in on a meeting between CBPR researchers and their community partners and observe the process. Then have them identify where they are in the research process and whether they adhered to CBPR principles during the meeting. What went well and what was challenging?

Questions

1. What questions should a researcher ask at each step of the research process in CBPR?

2. What are the skills that a CBPR researcher will need to enter into CBPR?

3. You have gotten a grant to conduct a CBPR project. However, it ended up taking more time than you expected to obtain the grant. During that time, the leader you were working with moved away. How would you re-engage the community?

❖ NOTES

1.   Break-out sessions. Taking It to the Curbside: Engaging Communities to Create Sustainable Change for Health. Conference, Boston, MA; April 2010.

2.   Hacker K, Chu J, Leung C, Marra R, Pirie A, Brahimi M, English M, Beckmann J, Acevedo-Garcia D, Marlin RP. The impact of Immigration and Customs Enforcement on immigrant health: perceptions of immigrants in Everett, Massachusetts, USA. *Social Science & Medicine*. 2011 Aug;73(4):586–94.

3.   Norris K, Brusuelas R, Jones L, Miranda J, Duru O, Mangione C. Partnering with community-based organizations: an academic institution's evolving perspective. *Ethnicity & Disease*. 2007;17(1):205.

4.   Baker EA, Homan S, Schonhoff R, Kreuter M. Principles of practice for academic/practice/community research partnerships. *American Journal of Preventive Medicine*. 1999 Apr;16(3 Suppl):86–93.

5.   Lawrence Mayor's Task Force. Tools for Research Partnerships in Lawrence, MA. Lawrence Mayor's Task Force, Lawrence, MA 2006; Available from: http://www.tuftsctsi.org/About-Us/CTSI-Components/Community-Engagement/~/media/B35A1D1535DB422D90E1A47544743E4E.ashx.

6.   Hacker K, Collins J, Gross-Young L, Almeida S, Burke N. Coping with youth suicide and overdose: one community's efforts to investigate, intervene, and prevent suicide contagion. *Crisis*. 2008;29(2):86–95.

7.   Institute for Community Health. *Policies.* Data confidentiality/IRB policy. Cambridge, MA: 2002. http://www.icommunityhealth.org/policies.html.

❖ RESOURCES

Community Campus Parternships for Health.http://www.ccph.info/.

6

Ethical Considerations
in CBPR

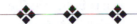

Members of the Havasupai tribe "had given DNA samples to university researchers starting in 1990, in the hope that they might provide genetic clues to the tribe's devastating rate of diabetes. But they learned that their blood samples had been used to study many other things, including mental illness and theories of the tribe's geographical origins that contradict their traditional stories." ... "I'm not against scientific research," said Carletta Tilousi, 39, a member of the Havasupai tribal council. "I just want it to be done right. They used our blood for all these studies, people got degrees and grants, and they never asked our permission."[1]

In the Havasupai case, biological samples were used for other purposes than those for which participant consent was given. This bioethical dilemma is one example of an ethical misstep that is pertinent to community-based research. In this scenario, the ethical dilemma occurred at both the individual as well as at the community level.

Not only was the consent of individuals who originally agreed to participate in the study for specific purposes disregarded, but there were implications for the entire community as well. In this chapter, we will explore some of the ethical issues encountered in CBPR. We will address the following areas:

1. Principles that guide ethical conduct of research and how they pertain to CBPR

2. The concepts of risk and benefit in CBPR

3. Ethical considerations unique to CBPR partnerships

❖ PRINCIPLES OF ETHICAL CONDUCT OF RESEARCH

The Belmont Report stands as a significant guidepost for the protection of human subjects and has influenced federal regulation and the conduct of biomedical and behavioral research nationally.[2] The report, issued in 1978, set out basic ethical principles underlying acceptable conduct of research involving human subjects. These include **respect for persons, beneficence**, and **justice.** Each of these principles has wide-ranging application for research involving individual human subjects. *Respect for persons* requires that the research is voluntary and that informed consent must be comprehensible to the individual. It also recognizes the protection of special populations of individuals with diminished autonomy, including children, prisoners, and those with cognitive disabilities. The concept of *beneficence* translates to protecting individuals from harm by minimizing risks and maximizing benefits. The concept of *justice* requires that the benefits and burdens of research are fairly distributed and relates to the selection of subjects in a manner that is just and fair. These concepts are the underpinnings of institutional review board (IRB) regulations. IRBs are the groups that oversee ethical conduct of research in academic environments.

There are a number of limitations of these guiding principles as they relate to CBPR. First, these concepts are primarily focused on the protection of the individual as research subject and not on the protection of communities as organized entities. Second, these principles lack guidelines for the ethical behavior of partners engaged in community/ academic collaboration. They also lack guidelines for assessing the risks and benefits to a community as a whole. In a recent review of

30 IRBs, Flicker and colleagues (2007) did not find adequate evidence that IRB policies and protocols applied to communities or to CBPR projects.[3] Today, as the practice of CBPR grows, we need to assess how the Belmont principles of respect, beneficence, and justice can be expanded to include communities in addition to the individuals residing within them.

In CBPR, there are several areas that deserve particular attention from an ethical standpoint.

1. Informed consent for research at the community level

2. Risks and benefits of research from a community perspective

3. Community standards of justice, including those of partnership ethics and economic distribution

❖ COMMUNITY INFORMED CONSENT

In human subjects research, informed consent involving any individual participant in research is required and must meet the standards set out in the Belmont Report. However, getting informed consent from an entire community is not realistic. So how does a researcher assess informed consent at the community level? How is the value of a research project communicated to the targeted community as a whole? Most importantly, how can a researcher feel confident that the research is perceived as acceptable and feasible to the community? Obtaining community consent is particularly challenging given that the individuals in the community are not homogeneous and opinions of various subgroups may differ substantially. To address these questions, CBPR researchers need to understand the values and mores of the community at large. They need to be aware of how these unstated perspectives pertain to ethical conduct in said community. Learning about the cultural perspectives, history, governance, and so forth of a community will help the researcher develop this understanding. Take, for example, the Havasupai tribe case, in which nonconsented research on DNA from blood samples suggested migration patterns that contradicted Havasupai origin myths. In addition, blood has great spiritual meaning to the Havasupai, and its return to the tribe brings ancestors home to their resting place. Thus, research using blood samples in this community raised additional ethical concerns about the care and appropriate return of samples to the tribe, none of which was considered.[1]

Community informed consent depends largely on defining and understanding the community of study and making sure that the leaders (formal and informal) support the research. In order to understand cultural considerations and assess the community's view of a research project, a CBPR researcher relies heavily on the community advisory board (CAB). The CAB serves as an entrée into the community. Its members provide needed advice and are the link between the researcher and the larger community. Their knowledge of the culture, local actors, politics, and social networks will help the researcher navigate the community landscape and determine project feasibility. As in the case of our Everett example, an actively engaged CAB that represents the community can be an enormous resource providing insight into acceptability of research and helping to ensure that there is community buy-in for the project. They will also be instrumental in helping the researcher understand the community context for the research (political and social climate), the competing priorities in the community that could limit participation, and the appropriateness of the chosen methods for consent and recruitment from both a cultural and practical standpoint. In our Everett example, the CAB was made up of leaders from the immigrant communities' advocacy groups. When we discussed recruitment, consent, and inclusion/exclusion criteria, the opinions of these individuals played an important role in decision making. CAB members who had access to constituents could therefore vet the project and the methods before we began and could tell us what would and would not work in their community. They translated the research tools, piloted them with immigrant groups, and led the recruitment efforts.[4] These community members were able to assess acceptability and feasibility and help researchers develop their eligibility criteria, their consent forms, and the informational materials used in recruitment. They reminded the research team of the need for low-literacy materials that were easily understood and nonthreatening. As researchers, we would not have been able to communicate our research goals to the community without the help of these leaders. In addition, these community partners were likely to take any findings from the project to future action.

To sum up, some of the critical questions to consider regarding community informed consent in CBPR include:

- Is the research project acceptable to the community of interest?
- Have you connected with leaders (informal and formal) to assess this acceptability?

- Have the criteria for inclusion been discussed with the community, and does this pose any ethical challenges?
- Are there particular cultural issues that need to be addressed?
- Is the CAB actively advising on these issues?

❖ RISKS AND BENEFITS FROM A COMMUNITY PERSPECTIVE

The concepts of risks and benefits from research at the individual level are easily understood; how will the research potentially benefit the participants and how will it potentially harm them? Most importantly, do the benefits outweigh the risks? In CBPR, not only will the researcher need to assess the individual risks and benefits of research, but he or she will need to understand the risks and benefits for the community as a whole. In other words, it is important to identify what the community will potentially gain or lose by participation in the research. Table 6.1 presents a framework for determining community

Table 6.1   Risk and Benefits of Research: Individual and Community Perspectives

	Risks /benefits of research process	Example	Risks/benefits of research outcomes	Example
Individual	Physical and psychosocial risks of the research interaction	Individual enrolls in a clinical trial for diabetes care. There are potential side effects from the medication during the trial (headaches, nausea, vomiting).	Physical and psychosocial risks of research findings	Individual may find that years after the research ends, unknown problems from the drug surface.
	Physical and psychosocial benefits of research interaction	Individual receives immediate relief from symptoms of illness.	Physical and psychosocial benefits of research findings	Individual may have his or her life extended if the research is successful.

(Continued)

Table 6.1   (Continued)

	Risks /benefits of research process	Example	Risks/benefits of research outcomes	Example
Community	Risks to group's structure and function because of engagement in research	The CAB has disagreement on the research project and the group structure breaks down as a result.	Risks to group's structure and function because of research findings	The research findings about high rates of asthma negatively stigmatize the community and lead to a decrease in property values.
	The community benefits structurally or functionally from the research process.	Community members gain new skills in the research process, and this increases community capacity and empowerment.	The community benefits structurally or functionally from the research results.	The findings shed positive light on the community, resulting in increased visibility and new resources from grants and press coverage.

risks/benefits compared to individual risks/benefits. This is discussed in greater detail in Ross and colleagues' (2010) work on human subjects protection in CBPR, from which this table was adapted.[5]

Community Risks and Benefits of the Research Process

Whereas an individual may experience physical or psychological risk from research, a community might experience a risk to its structure from the conduct or the results of research. From a risk perspective, the **process** of conducting CBPR may be stressful at both the individual and the community levels. Community members may have other priorities that compete for their attention, or they may have concerns about how recruitment is progressing. Similarly, the stress of CBPR on community-based organizations involved in research may also pose a risk. If the organization underestimates the time required or defers other responsibilities in favor of research, it could lead to organizational instability. There are also a myriad of other contextual forces facing communities, and during the research process, these priorities may be in direct conflict with the research process. For example, agreed-upon research methods such as random assignment or use of control groups may become untenable due to unforeseen political issues. In the face of sudden budget cuts impacting low-income women, a project that plans to randomly assign disadvantaged women to an intervention that offers additional support (navigation and coaching) may suddenly be seen as unjust or unethical because some people are excluded from receiving these services. The contextual community factors may ultimately force a mid-research shift in design. One study by Levy and colleagues (2006) speaks to this type of shift based on community values: that is, a random assignment of participants to an asthma intervention was planned, but due to community concerns, it was not possible. As Levy notes:

> Much CBPR research to date has been observational or otherwise fallen short of achieving clinical trial standards, which has potentially limited the impact of these studies on public health policy and programs. This may arise partly from the complexity of managing and sustaining equitable partnerships, as well as from resistance from community or city partners to aspects of scientific methodology that may not directly benefit the community in the short term (since a more rigorous methodology may conflict with addressing immediate needs).[6]

While there are community risks posed by the CBPR process, there are also a number of benefits to the community. Community members who are involved in CBPR are likely to learn new skills that contribute to increased community capacity for future problem solving. As community members gain facility with the use of data, research methodology, and systematic analysis, they are more likely to use evidence in their practice settings. In our Somerville example, community partners learned about surveillance strategies and data mapping. Since that time, not only have they continued to monitor data to assess suicide attempts and completions across the age range, but they have also used these skills to examine a host of community issues ranging from food security to youth development activities. The research process also builds new partnerships and alliances that could result in future collaborations for community good. Financial resources flow to the community during the research process, sup-porting community members. The research process in CBPR can also give voice to vulnerable populations as they are part of the decision-making process. The empowerment experience during CBPR as community members take on their own issues is a powerful tool in community development and organizing. Building leadership along with skills is perhaps one of the most significant outcomes of the CBPR process. In our Everett example, immigrant leaders had oppor-tunities to express themselves, shape the agenda, and lead efforts. Their empowerment is likely to translate to future action beyond the research agenda. Building capacity and empowerment in vulnerable communities is an important outcome of CBPR.

Community Risks and Benefits of the Research Results

Research **results** also have potential to pose risks as well as ben-efits for communities and community organizations involved in CBPR. An important ethical consideration is whether the research will con-tribute to local benefit or potentially cause harm. Certainly, results that help to solve local problems and garner support for action will likely be seen in a positive light and be embraced by community partners. However, community "harm" is also a possibility and is often unantici-pated. The results of research have the potential to stigmatize a com-munity or group if findings are disparaging. For example, in a study by Marcelli (2009) that surveyed various populations of immigrants, it was noted that one immigrant population was more likely to be undoc-umented than others.[7] This immigrant group perceived this type of information as stigmatizing and more likely to make them the target of law enforcement and deportation action. While this was not the intent of the research, it was an unforeseen outcome that put an already vul-nerable community at further risk. Other examples might include work on environmental issues that, while providing important evidence for health improvement, could also lead to loss of property values. Further, even neutral results could pose a risk to the community. For example, an evaluation of a community program that does not show effect could lead to loss of services to vulnerable populations and a concomitant loss of jobs for employees. Thus, it is important to discuss these ethical concerns with community partners at the beginning of a project. How will the community deal with unfavorable results? How will these be disseminated and translated to the community? How will they be utilized by both community and academic partners? How will the partnership protect the community without censoring findings?

Ethical Considerations for CBPR Partnerships

The CBPR academic/community **partnership** serves as the cornerstone for CBPR, and thus, it is important to understand the ethical considerations that shape and maintain these partnerships.[8] Partnership relies on power sharing in decision making, trust, respect, and economic distribution. But there are also risks and benefits inherent in being a community member of a research team. On one hand, there are the benefits of opportunities for skills acquisition and resources, while on the other hand, there are risks in that the relationship with academia may alter the community member's relationship with her or his own community. The person may even lose the respect of the community by becoming associated with the "outside" academics.[9] In addition, when the project is over and participants are no longer employed by the researcher, are they received back into the community? During the research process, there may also be conflicts among CAB members. These can lead to breakdown of the CAB and shifts in relationships that ultimately impact the community. For example, as a result of disagreement, community groups may fracture relationships with local government authorities, leading to problems within the community beyond the scope of the research project. Similarly, problems in relationships between researcher and community partners may arise if strategies for equitable sharing of power and economic resources are not in place. Does the project really allow for full participation of community partners? Is there adherence to the principles of CBPR? Are the constructs of partnership demonstrated in the research plan, in decision making, and in budgets? Researchers and their IRBs can help assess adherence to ethical principles in CBPR. As developed by the Community Engaged Research Subcommittee of the Harvard Catalyst Regulatory Core, a set of questions like the following can be helpful.[10]

- Does the proposed activity respond to the needs of this community and/or support existing infrastructure or networks?
- What is the plan for engaging with this community?
- How will the community be involved in the development and implementation of this particular project?

- What is the researchers' relationship with key stakeholders in the community?
- Has community risk versus individual risk been evaluated properly?
- Are recruitment strategies culturally/linguistically appropriate?
- What role will the community partner have in recruitment?
- How accessible/approachable is the researcher to the community stakeholders?
- Does the proposed consent form use (linguistically and culturally) appropriate language?
- Are there appropriate resources devoted to this project?
- What resources are required (financial, physical, etc.)?
- Is there an understanding of the institution's and community partners' needs/capacity for development and implementation of planned activities?
- Who will provide these resources?
- What is the community's role and expectation regarding the allocation of these resources?
- Are there financial resources available for translation services/interpreter services?

❖ DISSEMINATION

Part of the any CBPR project is dissemination of results, whether it be for publication in the scientific arena (peer-reviewed journals) or for action in the community-based context (discussion, forums, press releases). The manner in which CBPR dissemination is conducted is part of the discussion of risk and benefit to the community. Inappropriate dissemination in CBPR can have ethical implications. For example, if a community is not privy to research results or required to wait until "the paper comes out," this does not represent an equitable power-sharing relationship. While the lack of information may simply be an error of omission, it does not meet the requirements of a CBPR partnership. Thus, in CBPR, considerations for how the results will be communicated to the community should come first. The CAB should be involved in this discussion and in dissemination decision making. It needs to consider the best way to provide the results to the community, be that as a report, forum, newspaper article, or policy brief. Returning the findings to the community is a necessity, and it is this feedback loop that differentiates CBPR from other types of research. The use of the data for action is the major benefit for a community, and thus withholding the information would connote a risk. Worst-case scenarios are when the researcher disseminates results that the community partners are unaware of. Specific ethical questions around dissemination include:

- What plans/strategies are in place to disseminate the results and elicit feedback from community stakeholders?
- Will dissemination be through multiple venues (e.g., community forums, presentations, journal articles, websites)?
- Are these venues effective and accessible to both community members/providers and researchers?
- Will there be a process to inform community stakeholders about the role of the IRB?

❖ WHEN THE CBPR PROJECT ENDS

There may be ethical considerations that arise when a CBPR research project ends. Given the extensive community engagement in CBPR, this issue can be extremely important for the community and for the success of future academic/community partnerships. CBPR includes a focus on local action and sustainable change. The research is not just for research purposes but also has implications for local impact. A CBPR researcher must consider in all phases of the research the salient question of what the research will leave behind at the conclusion of a CBPR project. This may include direct impact from the research project and findings as well as the next steps following its conclusion. Toward that end, the CBPR partnership will have to grapple with questions of sustainability and how to obtain additional resources to support change and the activities associated with that change. Will the researcher continue to work with the community despite the loss of economic support (research grant funding)? Are the academic/community relationships ongoing or simply project based? Once a community group is mobilized and focused on action, questions about resources and sustainability will certainly arise, and the researchers must assess their role in this agenda. These are difficult questions to answer and perhaps are best assessed at the beginning of the project when the partnership determines its mutually agreed-upon goals. The use of MOAs or contractual agreements can certainly help, but the communication about these issues throughout the project is impera-tive. As in any relationship, the need for clear, ongoing communica-tion about difficult issues is something that the partnership must seek to address to avoid later confrontations and to plan for sustainability from the first day forward.

❖ CONCLUSION

The principles outlined in the Belmont Report of respect, beneficence, and justice are applicable not only to the individual involved in research but to communities as well. Part of being a CBPR practitioner is understanding how community risk and benefit are assessed and how it will affect your research design and dissemination. The impact of research may have long-term impact on communities that ranges far beyond the specific "side effects" of the research process. The CBPR researcher should consider the risks and benefits from the perspective of the individual and the community of interest. As IRBs assess CBPR, they too will need to consider the ethical implications of this type of work. A synopsis of these implications can be found in Table 6.2.

Table 6.2   Application of the Belmont Principles for CBPR

Informed Consent Voluntariness	• How is the community consent to be obtained? • How are community leaders and groups involved in recruitment? • What compensation is allocated to community members or groups? • What conflicts of interest may affect community participation?
Comprehension	• Are materials culturally and linguistically appropriate? • How are community leaders and groups involved in key decisions in the design and conduct of research? • What training will be provided to community members?
Risks and Benefits	• Individual • Individual by association with the group • Community • Disruption of community cohesion by research • Risks of disseminating sensitive data to the community • Risks of results harming community

Table 6.2	Continued
Selection of Subjects	• How is the community defined? • How are community leaders identified? • How are community leaders involved in defining inclusion and exclusion criteria? • What are the criteria for distribution of economic benefits? • How are community standards of fairness applied?

❖ QUESTIONS AND ACTIVITIES

Activities

Provide students with an example of a CBPR project that was conducted locally. Then have students point out potential ethical issues that this research might have raised for the individuals and the community.

A CBPR project focuses on environmental health hazards in a community of 80,000 people. The project is trying to assess the impact of an incinerator on cancer rates in the community. Based on preliminary findings, the community advisory board begins to suspect there is a link between the incinerator and higher cancer rates in one community. As the researcher, you have not drawn any conclusions yet or "crunched the data"; however, you are getting pressure from your community partners to release the data for advocacy purposes. Describe three ethical dilemmas that you might face given this situation.

Questions

1. What are the three concepts underpinning the Belmont Report? Describe each of these concepts.

2. How do these concepts apply to a community rather than an individual?

3. What are the risks of research when the community is the concern rather than an individual?

4. Are there times when an individual would be protected but a community might suffer harm? Describe an example of this.

5. What are some strategies a researcher could use to protect a community from hazardous research?

❖ NOTES

1.   Harmon A. Indian tribe wins fight to limit research of its DNA. *New York Times*. April 21, 2010.

2.   The National Commission for the Protection of Human Subjects of Biomedical and Behavioral Research. *The Belmont Report. Ethical Principles and Guideline for the Protection of Human Subjects of Research*. Washington, DC: U.S. Department of Health, Education, and Welfare; 1978.

3.   Flicker S, Travers R, Guta A, McDonald S, Meagher A. Ethical dilemmas in community-based participatory research: recommendations for institutional review boards. *Journal of Urban Health*. 2007 Jul;84(4):478–93.

4.   Hacker K, Chu J, Leung C, Marra R, Pirie A, Brahimi M, English M, Beckmann J, Acevedo-Garcia D, Marlin RP. The impact of Immigration and Customs Enforcement on immigrant health: perceptions of immigrants in Everett, Massachusetts, USA. *Social Science & Medicine*. 2011 Aug;73(4):586–94.

5.   Ross LF, Loup A, Nelson RM, Botkin JR, Kost R, Smith GR, Gehlert S. Human subjects protections in community-engaged research: a research ethics framework. *Journal of Empirical Research on Human Research Ethics: An International Journal*. 2010;5(1):5–18.

6.   Levy JI, Brugge D, Peters JL, Clougherty JE, Saddler SS. A community-based participatory research study of multifaceted in-home environmental interventions for pediatric asthmatics in public housing. *Social Science & Medicine*. 2006 Oct;63(8):2191–203.

7.   Marcelli E, Holmes L, Estella D, da Rocha F, Granberry P, Buxton O. *(In)Visible (Im)migrants: The Health and Socioeconomic integration of Brazilians in Metropolitan Boston*. San Diego, CA: Center for Behavioral and Community Health Studies, San Diego State University; 2009.

8.   Ross LF, Loup A, Nelson RM, Botkin JR, Kost R, Smith GR, Gehlert S. Nine key functions for a human subjects protection program for community-engaged research: points to consider. *Journal of Empirical Research on Human Research Ethics: An International Journal*. 2010;5(1):33–48.

9.   Minkler M, Wallerstein N., eds. *Comunity-Based Participatory Research for Health*. San Francisco, CA: Jossey-Bass; 2003.

10.   Harvard Catalyst Community Engaged Research (CeNR) Subcommittee. *Top Questions for IRB to Assess Community Engaged Research* (unpublished committee notes). Boston, MA: Harvard Catalyst; 2011.

7

Conclusions

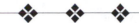

Community-based participatory research continues to expand as more communities and investigators understand the value of the approach. While the challenges are many, the rewards are great.

Throughout this book, I have reinforced the importance of the CBPR partnership between researcher and the community. CBPR is built on these relationships, which, when formed effectively, have the power to break down the barriers between academia and community and thereby improve the rapidity of evidence translation. The capacity built as a result of these partnerships can support community members to make data-driven decisions, evaluate their work, and catalyze change.

Developing and maintaining CBPR partnerships is in itself an important task for CBPR researchers. Can they adhere to the core values, including trust, respect, and equality? Can they strive to break down the power differentials between academics and community partners? When these partnerships succeed, they bring added value to the research and to both the researcher and the community. The community gains skills, evidence, and fuel for action; the researcher gains insight and inroads into the community, which changes the nature of the research process and supports the potential for community change. These insights will surely improve the relevancy of research and, ultimately, the potential for translation of evidence into practice. The findings of a CBPR project should align with the community's interest and provide beneficial information for action in an applied manner. CBPR strategies can bring us one step closer to engagement of communities as active players in the improvement of their own destiny. This is an important resource in our struggle to reduce disparities.[1]

❖ THE CBPR PROCESSES—STEP BY STEP

The CBPR process as described throughout the book can be broken down into a series of steps as outlined in Chapter 4 and provided here again in Table 7.1.

Table 7.1   Summary of CBPR Steps

Stage 1
Community Engagement[2-4]

- Identify the community of interest.
- Conduct a needs assessment to understand the issues for potential research.
- Meet the stakeholders.
- Develop relationships.
- Assemble a CAB.
- Choose an area for research.
- Conduct a literature review.
- Hone the research questions and hypotheses.

Stage 2
Research Design, Roles, and Responsibilities

- Discuss methods.
- Assess feasibility.
- Define roles for community and for researcher.
- Provide education and skill development.
- Conduct study.

Stage 3
Analysis, Interpretation, and Dissemination

- Assess skills.
- Develop iterative processes.
- Work with CAB for interpretation and context.
- Determine dissemination modes.
- Develop processes that allow all to participate.
- Identify action steps based on evidence.

These steps can be broken down into a variety of important concepts that are included in the following sections.

Community

As noted throughout this book, there are various elements of the CBPR process that a researcher should consider before, during, and after the research process. Starting with the identification of the community of interest, the researcher asks, "What is the community that I wish to engage? Who shall I partner with? Are my potential partners ready to engage?" To answer these questions, he or she must get to know the community under study, learn the actors, and understand the contextual factors surrounding them.

Engagement

The researcher then moves into the community engagement phase of CBPR in which he or she deepens relationships with identified community partners. These partnerships depend on mutual interest but rely on interpersonal skills to engender trust and share power. The researcher should ask what are the important issues facing their community partners. What are the questions that community members want to answer and for what purposes? More importantly, the researcher needs to demonstrate her or his value to the community. As in any valued relationship, there must be mutual benefit, trust, and value in the endeavor.

Defining the Questions

Refining the question from a broad community need to one that is focused and amenable to a research process is an important step that pulls from community knowledge and researcher skill. Once the research question is identified, hypotheses based on a jointly defined conceptual framework can be generated. From there, methods can be chosen. The researcher should ask how the problem is manifested. How is it operationalized? What are the potential solutions? What have people observed?

Choosing the Design and Methods

Choosing methods that are acceptable and feasible to the community while maintaining scientific rigor is a challenge in CBPR. The researcher and community members will need to assess the strengths and weaknesses of methods and ask pertinent questions. What are the limitations of any method from both a scientific and community perspective? Is it acceptable to the community? Will it provide a high level of evidence? Is it feasible in the community? What will the challenges be and how will we address them? Will it meet the needs of the community while meeting the needs of the researcher? Will it achieve validity and authenticity?

Conducting the Research

The research will require clarity between the partners as to who is doing what. Establishing these roles and responsibilities before fielding the research is imperative. So, too, there needs to be leadership to assure the timely completion of deliverables. The researcher needs to ask, who will collect the data? What training is needed? How will data move between partners? Are all the human subjects' protections in place? How are data stored and who will have access to the data?

The Analysis and Interpretation

At the beginning of the CBPR project, the CAB will need to determine how the analysis and interpretation should take place. The research team will likely take on the quantitative analysis, while community partners will likely be involved in interpretation. This is an extremely valuable benefit of the CBPR process. The interpretation of the data from the perspective of community partners often reveals unexpected concepts that reflect the realities of real life. The researcher must ask how the community partners want to be involved in analysis. What will be the loop for communication? How will community input be obtained?

Dissemination

As a CBPR project is completed and findings become ready for dissemination, community partners and researchers must jointly decide on two dissemination directions. What does the community want? How should findings be shared and with whom? Who will take the lead on community dissemination? Who will lead academic dissemination? How will authorship be established?

❖ THE CASE EXAMPLES: THE RESULTS

In each of the communities that were discussed in this book, CBPR has played a role in jump-starting community efforts for action. In addition, the findings from these projects have served the communities well while also providing generalizable information for other communities. The partnerships with local researchers remain and, in many cases, have turned their attention to other issues as problems have emerged.

Everett Immigrants

In the Everett immigrant health example, the CBPR project confirmed the observations of the CAB. Focus group and survey results revealed the following:

- Those in positions of authority—police, health care providers, health insurers—had power to interact with ICE and initiate deportation.
- Deportation fear had a negative effect at both the individual and communal levels.
  - Fear exacerbated chronic conditions: depression, high blood pressure, anxiety.
  - When immigrant communities do not trust their local institutions, it impacts their civic engagement.
- Primary care providers are witnessing the impact of deportation fear in their immigrant patients demonstrated by care avoidance, exacerbations of chronic medical conditions, and high levels of anxiety.

These results were shared with the larger community in a forum that provided an opportunity for community members from across the city to assess the data and have input into a set of recommendations. The first of these recommendations was to hold meetings with immigrants and the local police. Less than a year later, the police/immigrant relationships have been ongoing. Immigrant leaders report that police/immigrant relationships have greatly improved. Police are no longer arresting immigrants without driver's licenses. Rather, they are issuing citations, which do not require fingerprints. This action has alleviated stress within the community despite external anti-immigrant policies and procedures. Everett continues its work to fight racism and improve immigrant empowerment throughout the community.[5]

Somerville Youth Suicide

From 2001 to 2005, 19 young people died in Somerville from either suicide or overdose. The community had monitored the activity and, throughout the crisis, used data to design and launch a series of interventions. These action steps included a trauma response network, hiring a mental health coordinator at the health department, and funding a youth development program. In 2005, the last young person died from suicide/overdose, signaling an end to the contagion (Figure 7.1), and there have not been any subsequent deaths in this age group since that time. Data revealed that self-reported suicide attempts among high school students had dropped significantly (Figure 7.2).

Even though the suicide cluster ended, the city remains alert, maintains its mental health services, and monitors suicide activity.[6] The city has turned its attention to other issues, including obesity prevention and physical activity promotion. A host of other CBPR projects have since

Figure 7.1   Suicides and Lethal Overdoses Among 10-24-Year-Olds to, Somerville, Massachusetts, 1/2001–12/2005 (9 Suicides, 10 Overdoses)

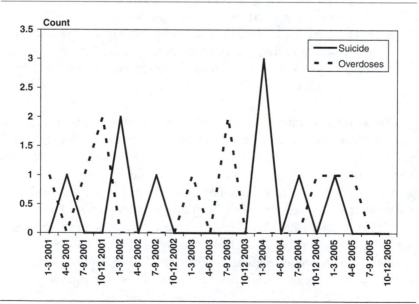

Source: Reproduced by permission from *Crisis*; Vol. 29(2): 86–95. © 2008 Hogrefe & Huber Publishers, www.hogrefe.com

Figure 7.2   High School Students Who Reported Suicidal Thoughts and
Behaviors in the Last 12 Months

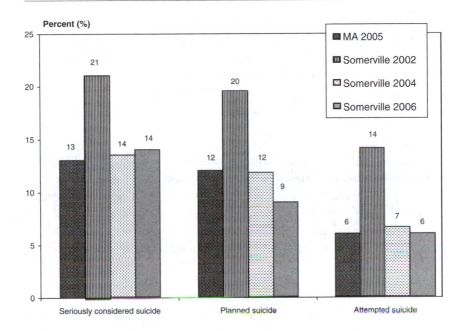

Data Source: MassCHIP v3.00r3.13 by January 2007, Somerville high school
2002 (N=1466), 2004 (N=1382), and 2006 (N=1003) health surveys.

Source: Reproduced by permission from *Crisis;* Vol. 29(2): 86–95. © 2008
Hogrefe & Huber Publishers, www.hogrefe.com

been launched, and the relationships between the city and surrounding
academics have flourished. More importantly, the city of Somerville has
become data driven, having built its own data capacity over time.

Cambridge BMI Disparities

In Cambridge, the BMI disparities project has only recently been
completed. A citywide report developed by the CBPR partners was
released and provides study findings. From retrospective data, the
project found the following:

- Obesity rates are similar for Black students whether or not their
  families qualified for free or reduced-price school meals.
- Among overweight or obese youth of all racial/ethnic groups,
  becoming fit helps them get to a healthy weight.
- The longer kids stay at a healthy weight when they are younger,
  the less likely they will become obese as adolescents.

In addition, to further highlight disparities, they found that Black students were significantly more likely to engage in obesigenic practices:

- 65% of Black males have at least two sugary drinks per day compared to 46% of all students.
- 41% of Black students watch more than 2 hours of TV on a school day compared to 29% of all students.
- 79% of Black girls did not meet physical activity guidelines compared to 69% of all students.

Interviews with Black parents and their children revealed that barriers to healthy living included lack of time to cook, to be active with kids, and to prepare fresh meals. In addition, social pressure to eat a certain way and frustration because nothing seems to work for weight loss added to the problem.

The CAB developed a set of recommendations that included the following:

- Involve the churches in promoting healthy lifestyles.
- Provide ongoing reinforcement of accurate nutrition education for both parents and kids.
- Make healthy food more accessible at corner stores.
- Have more community activities that promote family physical activity.

The CAB is actively looking for additional funding to bring these recommendations to fruition.[7]

In all three communities, CBPR has been a strategy for community members to ask and answer pressing questions. The relationships between researchers and community members have provided capacity and skills building, opened the door to future grants, and led the way to new ways of using data. Each phase of the CBPR process has associated benefits and challenges, as summarized in Table 7.2.

❖ THE FUTURE OF CBPR

CBPR is gaining popularity nationally in a variety of disciplines and across multiple topic areas. The number of CBPR publications is

Table 7.2 Critical Elements in CBPR[8]

| | CBPR Implementation and Potential Impact | | |
Research Element	CBPR Application	Community Benefits	Research Benefits	Research Challenges
Assembling a research team of collaborators with the potential for forming a research partnership	Identifying collaborators who are decision makers that can move the research project forward	Resources can be used more efficiently	Increases the probability of completing the research project as intended	Time to identify the right collaborators and convincing them that they play an important role in the research project
A structure for collaboration to guide decision making	Consensus on ethics and operating principles for the research partnership to follow, including protection of study participants	The beginning of building trust and the likelihood that procedures governing protection of study participants will be understood and acceptable	An opportunity to understand each collaborator's agenda, which may enhance recruitment and retention of study participants	An ongoing process throughout the life of research partnerships that requires skills in group facilitation, building consensus, and conflict accommodation
Defining the research question	Full participation of community in identifying issues of greatest importance; focus on community strengths as well as problems	Problems addressed are highly relevant to the study participants and other community members	Increased investment and commitment to the research process by participants	Time consuming; community may identify issues that differ from those identified by standard assessment procedures or for which funding is available

(Continued)

Table 7.2 (Continued)

		CBPR Implementation and Potential Impact		
Research Element	CBPR Application	Community Benefits	Research Benefits	Research Challenges
Grant proposal and funding	Community leaders/ members involved as a part of the proposal-writing process	Proposal is more likely to address issues of concern in a manner acceptable to community residents	Funding likelihood increases if community participation results in tangible indicators of support for recruitment and retention efforts, such as writing letters of support or serving on steering committee or as fiscal agents or co-investigators	Seeking input from the community may slow the process and complicate the proposal development effort when time constraints are often present
Research design	Researchers communicate the need for specific study design approaches and work with community to design more acceptable approaches, such as a delayed intervention for the control group	Participants feel as if they are contributing to the advancement of knowledge vs. as if they are passive research subjects and that a genuine benefit will be gained by their community	Community is less resentful of research process and more likely to participate	Design may be more expensive and/or take longer to implement; possible threats to scientific rigor
Participant recruitment and retention	Community representatives guide researchers to the most effective way to reach the intended study participants and keep them involved in the study	Those who may benefit most from the research are identified and recruited in a dignified manner rather than made to feel like research subjects	Facilitated participant recruitment and retention, which are among the major challenges in health research	Recruitment and retention approaches may be more complex, expensive, or time consuming

Formative data collection	Community members provide input to intervention design, barriers to recruitment and retention, etc., via focus groups, structured interviews, narratives, or other qualitative methods	Interventions and research approach are likely to be more acceptable to participants and thus of greater benefit to them and the broader population	Service-based and community-based interventions are likely to be more effective than if they are designed without prior formative data collection	Findings may indicate needed changes to proposed study design, intervention, and timeline, which may delay progress
Measures, instrument design, and data collection	Community representatives involved in extensive cognitive response and pilot testing of measurement instruments before beginning formal research	Measurement instruments less likely to be offensive or confusing to participants	Quality of data is likely to be superior in terms of reliability and validity	Time consuming; possible threats to scientific rigor
Intervention design and implementation	Community representatives involved with selecting the most appropriate intervention approach, given cultural and social factors and strengths of the community	Participants feel the intervention is designed for their needs while avoiding insult; provides resources for communities involved	Intervention design is more likely to be appropriate for the study population, thus increasing the likelihood of a positive study	Time consuming; hiring local staff may be less efficient than using study staff hired for the project

(Continued)

Table 7.2 (Continued)

	CBPR Implementation and Potential Impact			
Research Element	*CBPR Application*	*Community Benefits*	*Research Benefits*	*Research Challenges*
Data analysis and interpretation	Community members involved regarding their interpretation of the findings within the local social and cultural context	Community members who hear the results of the study are more likely to feel that the conclusions are accurate and sensitive	Researchers are less likely to be criticized for limited insight or cultural insensitivity	Interpretations of data by nonscientists may differ from those of scientists, calling for thoughtful negotiation
Manuscript preparation and research translation	Community members are included as coauthors of the manuscripts, presentations, newspaper articles, etc., following previously agreed-upon guidelines	Pride in accomplishment, experience with scientific writing, and potential for career advancement; findings are more likely to reach the larger community and increase potential for implementing or sustaining recommendations	The manuscript is more likely to reflect an accurate picture of the community environment of the study	Time consuming; requires extra mutual learning and negotiation

Source: Viswanathan M, Ammerman A, Eng E, Gartlehner G, Lohr KN, Griffith D, Rhodes S, Samuel-Hodge C, Maty S, Lux, L, Webb L, Sutton SF, Swinson T, Jackman A, Whitener L. *Community-Based Participatory Research: Assessing the Evidence.* Evidence Report/Technology Assessment No. 99 (Prepared by RTI–University of North Carolina Evidence-based Practice Center under Contract No. 290–02–0016). AHRQ Publication 04-E022- 2. Rockville, MD: Agency for Healthcare Research and Quality; 2004.

increasing annually from 4 in 2000 to more than 500 in 2010.[9] But the future of CBPR is dependent to a great extent on the benefits of the approach for both the community and the researcher. Does CBPR have the potential to build the partnerships necessary to produce innovative solutions grounded in practical experience?

Certainly, CBPR provides community partners with a nontraditional and hopefully more ethical approach to research intended to benefit both participants and the communities in which they live. Responding in part to a history of research exploitation, communities are now demanding to be more than "laboratories" for experiments.[10, 11] They want to engage, to shape, and, most importantly, to benefit in a very direct way from the research enterprise. In addition, community members want to examine the evidence and judge its applied value for themselves. CBPR therefore has enormous potential to improve both the translation of evidence into practice and the translation of practice into evidence. It has been touted as an approach to disparities research that engages and empowers vulnerable populations to alter their own destiny.[1, 12, 13] It is likely that as communities become activated, the demand for CBPR approaches and CBPR-competent researchers will increase.

National support in the form of funding opportunities, reports, and policy briefs also demonstrates the increasing interest in CBPR.[14–16] Foundations such as W.K. Kellogg and Robert Wood Johnson have identified CBPR as an important approach for community health research. The National Institutes of Health (NIH), the Centers for Disease Control and Prevention, and the U.S. Department of Health and Human Services have all incorporated CBPR into their requests for proposals.[17] The Clinical Translational Science Awards of the NIH have all incorporated community engagement as a core function[9] and have recently, along with other federal agencies, produced a book dedicated to the principles of community engagement.[2] The resources available for CBPR researchers are proliferating, with organizations wholly dedicated to its practice (Community Campus Partnerships for Health), online curricula, and listservs available for information sharing.[18] More recently, the language of CBPR has begun surfacing in health delivery system research in which providers and patients are being seen as important community partners.[19]

Yet while the opportunities for CBPR are increasing, there remains a gap in the number of researchers adequately trained in CBPR to meet the demand. The field is still rather young, and in most institutions, the number of interested students often outweighs the number of senior mentors. In addition, CBPR courses are not yet considered standard parts of graduate school curricula in fields such as health, education, psychology, social work, or sociology. Interested students are still challenged to find appropriate course offerings and available mentors to serve their needs and to introduce them to experiential learning opportunities in CBPR. More importantly, academic incentives related to CBPR in the promotion and tenure processes are often lacking or simply absent, which may discourage students from entering the field.

The growth of CBPR and its associated potential, however, may be self-limited if the field is unable to concretely describe and demonstrate the benefits of this approach. Lingering questions need to have answers. Does CBPR really improve science (relevancy, authenticity, recruitment, retention)? Can CBPR employ the highest-quality science while adhering to CBPR principles (experimental design)? Does CBPR speed the translational process? Does it lead to community improvements in health, education, and social services? Can the results of CBPR in one community be generalized to other communities? What are the contextual factors that determine cross-population generalizability in CBPR? As noted in the recent Agency for Health Care Research and Quality (AHRQ) report, "An inherent challenge faced by anyone trying to evaluate the quality and impact of CBPR methodology is the fact that being true to the methods makes it nearly impossible to compare CBPR rigorously to research carried out with more traditional research methods."[8]

As noted in Table 7.2, CBPR has many advantages over traditional research. It provides a host of benefits directly to the community, including resources, skills, respect, and access to knowledge. For the researcher, it facilitates recruitment and retention of hard-to-reach populations, provides a high level of relevancy, and lends community interpretation and meaning that improves validity and authenticity. However, CBPR has it challenges as well, ranging from the time required to design complexity and lack of control. Today, as the field matures, CBPR investigators are employing more rigorous scientific methods, and with that progress, there is an increasing understanding of why and when to utilize a CBPR approach based on its advantages and disadvantages. For example, CBPR may be particularly well suited for research on disparities and social determinants of health, while it may be poorly suited for clinical drug trials. It may lend itself to formative and exploratory research more than to randomized intervention studies. As we move forward with CBPR, we will need to attune ourselves to the best applications of the approach that will yield the highest return.

Finally, CBPR should be judged not only on the quality of the science but also on its ability to improve academic/community relationships, to contribute to community capacity building and to result in sustainable community change. While these outcomes may not typically be considered legitimate research outcomes, in CBPR, they are a significant result of the process for both academic and community partners. In the pursuit of community health and welfare improvement, communities must be empowered to catalyze, deliver, and ultimately sustain change. CBPR is one approach that enables this ultimate goal.

❖ RESOURCES

- Community Campus Partnerships for Health

   http://www.ccph.info/
   http://www.cbprcurriculum.info/

- Viswanathan M, Ammerman A, Eng E, Gartlehner G, Lohr KN, Griffith D, Rhodes S, Samuel-Hodge C, Maty S, Lux, L, Webb L, Sutton SF, Swinson T, Jackman A, Whitener L. *Community-Based Participatory Research: Assessing the Evidence.* Evidence Report/Technology Assessment No. 99 (Prepared by RTI–University of North Carolina Evidence-based Practice Center). AHRQ Publication 04-E022-2. Rockville, MD: Agency for Healthcare Research and Quality; July 2004.
- Clinical and Translational Science Awards Consortium. Communtiy Engagement Key Function Committee Task Force on the Principles of Community Engagement. *Principles of Community Engagement*, 2nd ed. Rockville, MD: NIH; 2011.
- Fleischer, MA (ed.). *Community-Engaged Research: A Quick Start for Researchers.* http://ctsi.ucsf.edu/files/CE/guide_for_researchers.pdf. CTSI at UCSF; 2010.

❖ NOTES

1. Wallerstein NB, Duran B. Using community-based participatory research to address health disparities. *Health Promotion & Practice.* 2006 Jul;7(3):312–23.

2. Clinical and Translational Science Awards Consortium. Communtiy Engagement Key Function Committee Task Force on the Principles of Community Engagement. *Principles of Community Engagement,* 2nd ed. Rockville, MD: NIH; 2011.

3. Israel BA, Parker EA, Rowe Z, Salvatore A, Minkler M, Lopez J, Butz A, Mosley A, Coates L, Lambert G, Potito PA, Brenner B, Rivera M, Romero H, Thompson B, Coronado G, Halstead S. Community-based participatory research: lessons learned from the Centers for Children's Environmental Health and Disease Prevention Research. *Environmental Health Perspectives.* 2005 Oct;113(10):1463–71.

4. Minkler M, Wallerstein N, eds. *Comunity-Based Participatory Research for Health.* San Francisco, CA: Jossey-Bass; 2003.

5. Hacker K, Chu J, Leung C, Marra R, Pirie A, Brahimi M, English M, Beckmann J, Acevedo-Garcia D, Marlin RP. The impact of Immigration and Customs Enforcement on immigrant health: perceptions of immigrants in Everett, Massachusetts, USA. *Social Science & Medicine.* 2011 Aug;73(4):586–94.

6. Hacker K, Collins J, Gross-Young L, Almeida S, Burke N. Coping with youth suicide and overdose: one community's efforts to investigate, intervene, and prevent suicide contagion. *Crisis.* 2008;29(2):86–95.

7. Chomitz V, Arsenault L, Banks C, et al. *H.E.L.P. Culminating Report.* Cambridge, MA: Institute for Community Health; 2011.

8. Viswanathan M, Ammerman A, Eng E, Gartlehner G, Lohr KN, Griffith D, Rhodes S, Samuel- Hodge C, Maty S, Lux, L, Webb L, Sutton SF, Swinson T, Jackman A, Whitener L. *Community-Based Participatory Research: Assessing the Evidence.* Evidence Report/Technology Assessment No. 99 (Prepared by RTI–University of North Carolina Evidence-based Practice Center). AHRQ Publication 04-E022-2. Rockville, MD: Agency for Healthcare Research and Quality; July 2004.

9. Blumenthal DS. Is community-based participatory research possible? *American Journal of Preventive Medicine.* 2011 Mar;40(3):386–9.

10. Gamble VN. Under the shadow of Tuskegee: African Americans and health care. *American Journal of Public Health.* 1997 Nov;87(11):1773–8.

11. Malone RE, Yerger VB, McGruder C, Froelicher E. "It's like Tuskegee in reverse": a case study of ethical tensions in institutional review board review of community-based participatory research. *American Journal of Public Health.* 2006 Nov;96(11):1914–9.

12. Chung B, Jones L, Terry C, Jones A, Forge N, Norris KC. Story of Stone Soup: a recipe to improve health disparities. *Ethnitcy & Disease*. 2010;20(1 Suppl 2):S2–9–14.

13. Israel BA, Coombe CM, Cheezum RR, et al. Community-based participatory research: a capacity-building approach for policy advocacy aimed at eliminating health disparities. *American Journal of Public Health*. 2010;100(11):2094–102.

14. Minkler M, Blackwell AG, Thompson M, Tamir H. Community-based participatory research: implications for public health funding. *American Journal of Public Health*. 2003 Aug;93(8):1210–3.

15. George MA, Daniel M, Green LW. Appraising and funding participatory research in health promotion. 1998–99. *International Quarterly of Community Health Education*. 2006;26(2):171–87.

16. Seifer SD, Kauper-Brown J, Robbins A. *Directory of Funding Sources for Community-based Participatory Research Conference on Improving the Health of Our Communities Through Collaborative Research; June 28–30, 2004*. Portland, OR: Community-Campus Partnerships for Health; 2004.

17. Faridi Z, Grunbaum JA, Gray BS, Franks A, Simoes E. Community-based participatory research: necessary next steps. *Preventing Chronic Disease*. 2007 Jul;4(3):A70.

18. Community-Campus Partnerships for Health. Seattle, WA. http://www.ccph.info/.

19. Patient-Centered Outcomes Research Institute (PCORI). Washington, DC. http://www.pcori.org/.

About the Author

Dr. Karen Hacker is the executive director of the Institute for Community Health in Cambridge, Massachusetts. She is also an associate professor of medicine at the Harvard Medical School and Harvard School of Public Health, where she teaches "Community-Based Participatory Action Research." She serves as the Senior Medical Director for Public and Community Health at the Cambridge Health Alliance and provides leadership for population health initiatives as well as practicing as a primary care physician. She received her M.D. from Northwestern University, her adolescent medicine fellowship from Children's Hospital of Los Angeles, and her master's from Boston University. She has extensive experience with CBPR and has worked with diverse community partners on topics that include child mental health, immigrant health, obesity prevention, and school health centers. She has authored and co-authored numerous journal articles and research reports, served on numerous state and national committees, and led CBPR efforts for the Harvard Clinical and Translational Award-Harvard Catalyst.

⊛SAGE research**methods**

The essential online tool for researchers from the world's leading methods publisher

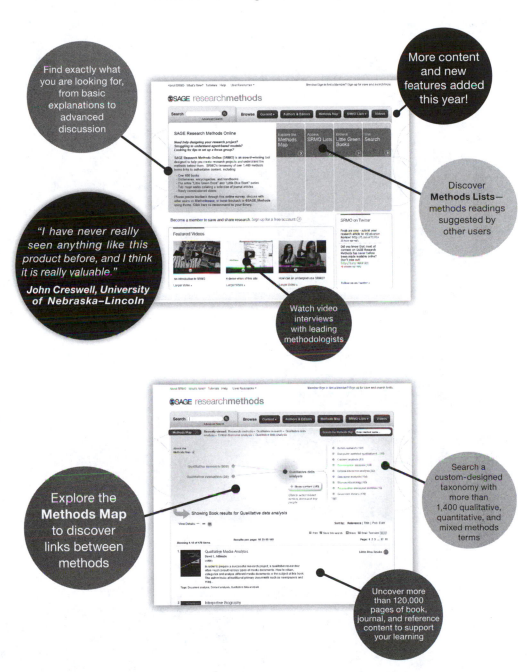

Find exactly what you are looking for, from basic explanations to advanced discussion

More content and new features added this year!

"I have never really seen anything like this product before, and I think it is really valuable."

John Creswell, University of Nebraska–Lincoln

Discover **Methods Lists**— methods readings suggested by other users

Watch video interviews with leading methodologists

Explore the **Methods Map** to discover links between methods

Search a custom-designed taxonomy with more than 1,400 qualitative, quantitative, and mixed methods terms

Uncover more than 120,000 pages of book, journal, and reference content to support your learning

Find out more at
www.sageresearchmethods.com